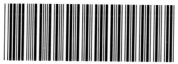

Cancer Grading Manual

Ivan Damjanov • Fang Fan

Editors

Cancer Grading Manual

Second Edition

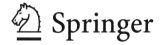 Springer

Editors

Ivan Damjanov, M.D., Ph.D.
Department of Pathology
The University of Kansas
School of Medicine
Kansas City, KS
USA

Fang Fan, M.D., Ph.D.
Department of Pathology
The University of Kansas
School of Medicine
Kansas City, KS
USA

ISBN 978-3-642-34515-9   ISBN 978-3-642-34516-6   (eBook)
DOI 10.1007/978-3-642-34516-6
Springer Heidelberg New York Dordrecht London

Library of Congress Control Number: 2013933010

Printed on acid-free paper

Springer is part of Springer Science+Business Media (www.springer.com)

Preface to the Second Edition

It is hard to believe that 5 years have passed from the time the first edition of this manual was published in 2007. In the meantime, we have heard a lot of comments about our book, both positive and critical, as well as suggestions on how to make it more user-friendly and useful. Finally, after a discussion with the publisher, we concluded that there is a real need for an updated version of our grading book. Thus, we undertook the task of updating the first edition, adding new things wherever needed, and modifying other parts in concordance with the new developments in diagnostic pathology.

For the second edition, we have retained most of the features of the first edition, especially those pertaining to the layout, which many readers liked. The format of the book was reduced to make it more handy and comparable to the *AJCC Staging Manual*, so that these two books could be used in tandem. We hope that readers of the previous edition will like the newly introduced changes, and we also trust that the new readers will find them useful as well.

This book is meant to be a manual and a quick reference for surgical pathologists and their trainees—a compact single volume designed for consultation rather than for systematic reading. We hope that the reader will like our commentaries, practical suggestions, and practice-proven know-how advice, tips, and hints. In the book, we have included answers to some common questions, guidance on how to do the grading, which tumors to grade and which not. We hope that the illustrations will amplify our written message and explain things that are hard to formulate in simple sentences.

At the end of the preface to the first edition, we have invited the readers to send us their comments, and we thank all those who did so. We would love to hear from readers of the second edition as well by e-mail (idamjano@kumc.edu or ffan@kumc.edu) or in any other form.

Ivan Damjanov, M.D., Ph.D.
Fang Fan, M.D., Ph.D.

Preface to the First Edition

The grading and staging of tumors are routinely performed during the work-up of most patients who have cancer. Whereas the staging of tumors relies on a wealth of clinical, intraoperative, or radiologic data, tumor grading remains in the domain of pathologists—hence, the idea to compile a book for our colleagues in diagnostic surgical pathology and their residents.

Like most surgical pathologists, we grade and stage tumors every day, and the assigned values are included in the final pathology reports. During the sign-out, we use the *AJCC Cancer Staging Handbook* or *TNM Atlas: Illustrated Guide to the TNM Classification of Malignant Tumors.* As strange as it might sound, although many textbooks contain instructions on how to grade tumors, there is no concise, "ready-to-use," practice-oriented manual on the microscopic grading of tumors. Confronted with the perceived need for such a book (and especially encouraged by our residents), we undertook the task of extracting the pertinent facts from books, monographs, and seminal papers and presenting them in a concise form. Since pathology is a visual discipline, the publisher allowed us to liberally use color microphotographs whenever needed to make a point and thus produce an illustrated manual that could be applied in the daily practice of surgical pathology without the need to resort to other books. We thank the publisher for this support. From now on, our residents will no longer need to ask us which book they should use for grading tumors. We hope that other practicing surgical pathologists will find the book useful as well and keep it as a companion to their favorite tumor staging manual.

In preparing this book, we have consulted a number of leading textbooks of surgical pathology, monographs prepared by the experts of the World Health Organization, and tumor atlases published by the Armed Forces Institute of Pathology. Readers interested in these sources, as well the recent comprehensive, seminal articles, will find them listed as references at the end of each chapter. While there is nothing new in this compilation, it is the first to present these data in such a condensed form, illustrated with so many color images.

We have concentrated on tumors that are common and thus have omitted some of the less common neoplasms and some of the neoplastic diseases that are in the domain of subspecialties of pathology (most notably hematology). We have not included the grading of some common inflammatory nonneoplastic diseases, such as chronic hepatitis or lupus nephritis. We hope that readers will not mind, but if you feel that some omissions are unpardonable, we would love to hear from you. Comments and suggestions for improvements, updates, or revisions are welcome.

Ivan Damjanov, M.D., Ph.D.
Fang Fan, M.D., Ph.D.

Contents

Contributors

Karen L. Chang, M.D. Department of Pathology, Kaiser Permanente Southern California, Los Angeles, CA, USA

Liang Cheng, M.D. Department of Pathology and Laboratory Medicine, Indiana University School of Medicine, Indianapolis, IN, USA

Ivan Damjanov, M.D., Ph.D. Department of Pathology, The University of Kansas School of Medicine, Kansas City, KS, USA

Fang Fan, M.D., Ph.D. Department of Pathology, The University of Kansas School of Medicine, Kansas City, KS, USA

John F. Fetsch, M.D. Soft Tissue Pathology, The Joint Pathology Center, Silver Spring, MD, USA

Garth R. Fraga, M.D. Department of Pathology, The University of Kansas School of Medicine, Kansas City, KS, USA

Nina Gale, M.D. Faculty of Medicine, Institute of Pathology, University of Ljubljana, Ljubljana, Slovenia

Zoran Gatalica, M.D., D.Sc. Department of Pathology, Creighton University School of Medicine, Omaha, NE, USA

Caris Life Sciences, Phoenix, AZ, USA

Robert M. Genta, M.D. University of Texas Southwestern Health Science Center at Dallas and Miraca Life Sciences, Dallas, TX, USA

Antonio Lopez-Beltran, M.D., Ph.D. Department of Surgery, Unit of Anatomic Pathology, Cordoba University School of Medicine, Cordoba, Spain

Muchou Joe Ma, M.D., Ph.D. Department of Pathology (Center for Diagnostic Pathology), Florida Hospital Orlando, Orlando, FL, USA

Gregory T. MacLennan, M.D. Institute of Pathology, Case Western Reserve University, Cleveland, OH, USA

Markku Miettinen, M.D. National Cancer Institute, Bethesda, MD, USA

Cesar Moran, M.D. Department of Pathology, University of Texas, M.D. Anderson Cancer Center, Houston, TX, USA

William L. Neumann, M.D. University of Texas Southwestern Health Science Center at Dallas and Miraca Life Sciences, Dallas, TX, USA

Jaime Prat, M.D., Ph.D., FRCPath Department of Pathology, Hospital de la Santa Creu i Sant Pau, Autonomous University of Barcelona, Barcelona, Spain

Nagarjun Rao, M.D. Department of Pathology, Medical College of Wisconsin, Milwaukee, WI, USA

Saul Suster, M.D. Department of Pathology, Medical College of Wisconsin, Milwaukee, WI, USA

Lawrence M. Weiss, M.D. Department of Pathology, Clarient Pathologist Services, Inc., Aliso Viejo, CA, USA

Ming Zhou, M.D., Ph.D. Surgical Pathology and Urologic Pathology, NYU Medical Center Tisch Hospital, New York, NY, USA

Nina Zidar, M.D. Faculty of Medicine, Institute of Pathology, University of Ljubljana, Ljubljana, Slovenia

History and General Aspects of Tumor Grading

Ivan Damjanov

Malignity only differs in degree.
Rudolph Virchow, 1860

1.1 History of Tumor Grading

The relationship between the tumor morphology and the clinical behavior of tumors has been known since the early studies of Rudolf Virchow (1821–1902) and the scientific beginnings of microscopic pathology. From the historical point of view, however, the first attempts to correlate the microscopic features of tumors with their biology and clinical behavior are traditionally attributed to David Paul von Hansemann (1858–1920) [1–3]. This German pathologist, who was a student of Virchow, studied systematically the microscopic pathology of tumors and in the 1890s published his pioneering observations on abnormal mitotic figures. He also introduced the terms *anaplasia* and *dedifferentiation* (German: *Entdifferenzirung*) and was the first to suggest that the clinical behavior of tumors could be predicted from their microscopic characteristics. His novel observations on microscopic tumor cell atypia, anaplasia, and asymmetrical mitoses were summarized in an 1897 book [3]. Von Hansemann's teaching and his book were at that time considered revolutionary and quite controversial, stimulating many scientific discussions [4]. Nevertheless, the book was apparently widely read, and it reappeared 5 years later in its second edition (Fig. 1.1). In contrast to many theoretical textbooks dominating the field of pathology, this treaty was based on meticulous microscopic study of tumors and could be considered "evidence based." It was illustrated with original drawings supporting the author's views of cancer (Fig. 1.2). The clarity of these illustrations is fascinating even today.

In the 1920s, Albert C. Broders of the Mayo Clinic pathology staff published his experience with grading of squamous cell carcinoma of the lip and skin and correlated the histologic grade with the outcome of the of the neoplastic disease in patients harboring these tumors (Fig. 1.3) [5, 6]. Broders implied that all malignant tumors could be divided into four groups, depending on the extent of tumor cell differentiation. He used a four-tiered system and classified tumors into those that contain 25, 50, 75 or 100 % incompletely differentiated of the cells. His ideas on grading of tumors were subsequently adopted by many others and applied to tumors in other organ systems.

Greenough was the first to propose the idea of histologic grading for breast cancers in 1925 [7]. He and his colleagues assigned a grade to tumors based on the overall evaluation of eight histologic features. Using a three-tiered grading system, these authors showed a clear association between tumor grade and the 5-year "cure" in their clinical-pathologic study. It is fair to say that all the current breast grading systems stem from his original ideas and the work from the early twentieth century.

I. Damjanov, M.D., Ph.D.
Department of Pathology,
The University of Kansas School of Medicine,
Kansas City, KS, USA
e-mail: idamjano@kumc.edu

I. Damjanov, F. Fan (eds.), *Cancer Grading Manual*,
DOI 10.1007/978-3-642-34516-6_1, © Springer-Verlag Berlin Heidelberg 2013

Die

mikroskopische Diagnose

der

bösartigen Geschwülste

von

Professor Dr. **David von Hansemann.**

Zweite Auflage.

Mit 106 Figuren im Text.

Berlin 1902.

Verlag von August Hirschwald.

N.W. Unter den Linden 68.

Fig. 1.1 Front page of the second edition of von Hansemann's textbook

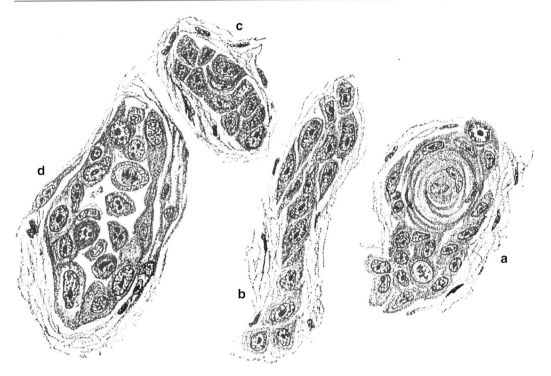

Fig. 1.2 Artist's drawing of squamous carcinoma cells (From Von Hansemann D (1902) Die mikroskopische Diagnose der bösartigen Geschwülste, 2nd edn. A. Hirschwald, Berlin)

The concepts and conclusions drawn from these early studies have been used and modified repeatedly during the following years [8–10]. Some of the early students of grading combined it with staging, and their eponymous systems, such as the Dukes system for classifying colonic cancer [8], survived up to modern times. For breast cancer alone, more than 10 grading methods and their modifications have been proposed. By the late 1990s, over 40 histologic grading systems for prostatic carcinoma were proposed [11].

Despite a plethora of longitudinal retrospective and prospective studies showing the usefulness of microscopic grading, the idea of routine tumor grading did not gain much popularity among clinicians and pathologists up to 1970s. This was partly due to the complexity and subjectivity of some grading systems and partly due to the limitation of treatment options corresponding to different grades of the tumor. However, as the treatment options multiplied, the need for better stratification of patients became imperative.

Carriaga and Henson [12] found that the overall frequency of grading increased over the 15-year period of 1973–1987 by 18 % for all sites combined: 65 % of all cancers were graded in 1983–1987, compared with 47 % in 1973–1977.

Today there is an overwhelming consensus that tumor grading has in many instances not only a prognostic value, but also it might have a significant impact for choosing optimal treatment for particular tumors (predictive value).

1.2   General Principles of Tumor Grading

The main principle of tumor grading, originating from Broders' earlier work, is to identify parts of the tumor that are differentiated and express the extent of differentiation as a percentage of the entire tumor. The grading method is to use standard light microscopic interpretation of hematoxylin and eosin (H&E)-stained tissue sections. Some earlier grading

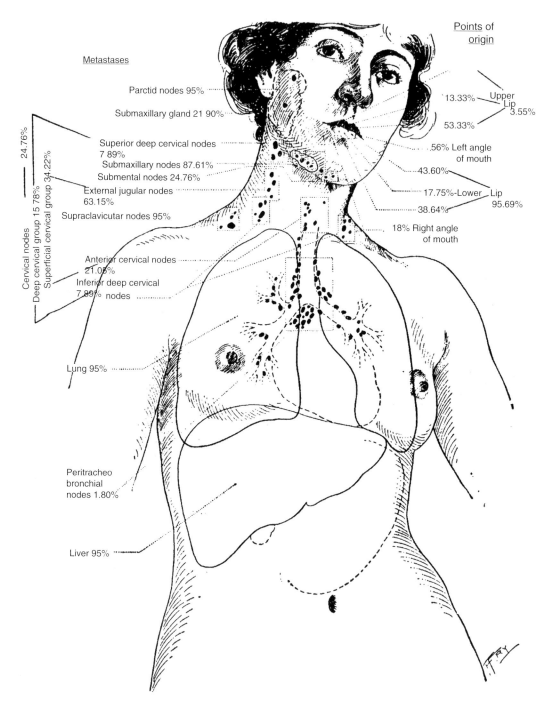

Fig. 1.3 Broders' seminal paper on grading of tumors (Broders [5])

systems required grading of up to 15 histologic features which included grading of growth pattern, cell morphology, and tumor stromal response [13]. Such elaborate systems were found to be, however, cumbersome, unreliable, and not always reproducible. Therefore, a good grading scheme should be simple, easy to perform, reliable, and reproducible and should be able to pass the test of time and prove to be clinically useful [14].

The grading process in general includes assessment of both the architectural and cytologic features of a tumor. Some grading systems focus, however, mainly on one histologic feature. For example, grading of prostatic adenocarcinoma is based entirely on the architecture feature, and grading of renal cell carcinomas is based entirely on their nuclear features. In general, the most poorly differentiated part of the tumor determines the final tumor grade, with the exception of the Gleason grading system for prostatic adenocarcinoma in which the two most prevalent patterns are used for grading. It is worth mentioning, however, that even such well-established systems as the Gleason grading of prostate carcinoma are still being modified; a need for the identifying a tertiary pattern has been formulated, and the reporting of cancer grades was found to vary even among the urologic pathologists [15, 16].

So far, all grading systems are designed for grading the primary untreated tumor. Attempts have been made to apply the same grading scheme for metastatic foci and residual tumors after radiation and/or chemotherapy. Currently, there is no general consensus on this issue.

1.3   Ancillary Methods Used in Tumor Grading

Almost all systems for grading of malignant tumors are currently based on morphologic evaluation of tumor sections under the microscope. Several improvements of the time-honored microscopic approach have been recommended, but few of these have been adopted in routine surgical pathology practice. Probably the most notable exception is the immunohistochemical staining with the antibody MIB-1 (Ki-67), recognizing cell proliferation. This immunohistochemical technique has been proposed as an objective supplement of several tumor-grading systems, including the grading of breast carcinoma, brain astrocytoma, and lymphoma [17, 18]. It is expected that with advanced understanding of diseases and development of new technology,

prognostic biomarkers and genetic information may be incorporated in tumor grading in the future.

The prognostic and predictive value of microscopic tumor grading can be enhanced by using other immunohistochemical methods [17–21]. For example, in breast carcinoma, immunohistochemical data with antibodies to estrogen receptor, bcl-2 gene product, and Her2/neu have predictive value in both univariate and multivariate analysis and are useful for predicting the patients' response to specific therapy [18]. In most instances however, there is no consensus on the value of these ancillary methods. For example, the International Consensus Panel on cytology and bladder tumor markers could not agree on the value of multiple markers in predicting tumor recurrence, progression, metastasis, or response to therapy [19]. This Panel evaluated various prognostic indicators and classified them into six groups:

- Microsatellite-associated markers
- Proto-oncogenes/oncogenes
- Tumor suppressor genes
- Cell cycle regulators
- Angiogenesis-related factors
- Extracellular matrix adhesion molecules

The members of the Panel concluded that certain markers, such as Ki-67 and p53, appear to be promising in predicting recurrence and progression of bladder cancer, but the data are still incomplete. It was also concluded that no consensus should be attempted until major prospective studies are performed and definitive criteria for test positivity are defined. Further recommendation included performing studies of clearly defined patient populations, standardization of techniques for evaluating the markers, and clearly specified clinical endpoints with good statistical documentation.

The use of ancillary methods has been especially championed by the neuropathologists who have used several techniques to estimate the proliferative potential of brain tumors. As summarized in a recent review article by Quinones-Hinojosa [21] in addition to immunohistochemical staining with antibody Ki-67 (MIB-1), such measurements can include bromodeoxyuridine labeling index (BrdU LI), flow cytometry (FCM), and staining for the proliferating cell nuclear antigen (PCNA) and argyrophilic nucleolar organizing regions (AgNOR). At the present time, MIB-1 and AgNOR are the simplest and most reliable of these techniques. Radiographic studies such as positron emission tomography (PET), single photon emission computed tomography (SPECT), and most recently magnetic resonance spectroscopy (MRS) used as follow-up measures have the potential to provide an assessment of tumor proliferation without the need for invasive measures.

data, one may construct nomograms which may predict the outcome of the treatment, disease-free survival, or cure rate. This may be true for many epithelial tumors, brain tumors, as well as sarcomas of bones and soft tissues, even though many tumors still do not lend themselves to grading [22, 23]. Nevertheless, most tumors can be stratified microscopically, and if the grade assigned to them is combined with grading and other clinical data, it may serve as a powerful predictor of clinical outcome of neoplastic disease, as well as for choosing the appropriate therapy for many cancer patients.

1.4   Clinical Value of Tumor Grading

Data obtained by tumor grading are usually combined with those obtained by tumor staging and other clinical approaches and are then evaluated by multivariate analysis. In most studies of this kind, it has been shown that tumor grade contributes to the multivariate prognosis, but in some, it was shown that the grading could be in itself a valid prognosticator even in a univariate analysis. Henson [9] in 1988 published a study on the relation between tumor grade and patient outcome. More than 500,000 cases from 15 anatomic sites with up to 9-year follow-up were reviewed. The results showed that stage by stage, the grade further subdivided the overall survival rates for each site into distinct subsets that were significantly different. Carriaga and Henson [12] later performed a similar study and demonstrated that the histologic grade is a strong predictor of outcome that refines the prognostic information provided by the stage of disease. There are numerous other studies reported in the literature showing that microscopic tumor grading has independent prognostic value [14–17].

Due to the availability of different treatment options, tumor grading now has an additional clinical value as guidance for therapy choice. While surgical resection may suffice for a low-grade tumor, additional radiation and/or chemotherapy may be necessary for high-grade tumors. By combining grading with staging and clinical

1.5   Perspective

Grading of tumors has been an integral part of the pathologic examination of biopsies and surgically resected tumors for close to 100 years. During that period, numerous studies have been performed on the value of grading, and numerous modifications of various systems have been proposed and tested. Grading of tumors could be thus considered as a work in progress, and additional efforts to improve the existing schemes are obviously necessary. This will require additional prospective studies, improvement of the intra- and interobserver variability, statistical evaluation of reproducibility, and correlation with the end-point treatment outcome results.

Current systems for grading tumors are far from perfect and ideal. New modifications of old systems are constantly tested, and many improvements are reported, often validated in practice or reviewed in view of the contributions of the new technologies [23, 24]. Controversies persist, but still, the general consensus of pathologists, surgeons, and clinical oncologists is that the tumor grades deserve to be part of routine pathology reports for most tumors and should be performed by diagnostic pathologists as meticulously as the situation requires [25]. In concordance with this approach, the Association of Directors of Anatomic and Surgical Pathology (ADASP) also recommended that tumor grades be included in standardized surgical pathology reports, implying that such reporting could contribute positively to patient care [26]. Although there are still no universal position papers on the use of modern technologies, intuitively, most of us also believe that the technologic advances in the field of molecular and cancer cell biology will significantly contribute to the grading of tumors and make it even more clinically relevant than ever before.

References

1. von Hansemann D (1890) Über assymentrische Zellteilung in Epithelkrebsen und deren biologische Bedeutung [Asymmetric cell division in epithelial cancer and its biological meaning.]. Virchows Arch Pathol Anat Histopathol 119:299–326
2. von Hansemann D (1892) Über die Anaplasie des Geschwülstzellen und die assymetrische Mitose [Anaplasia of tumor cells and asymmetric mitosis.]. Virchows Arch Pathol Anat Histopathol 121:436–449
3. von Hansemann D (1897) Die mikroskopische Diagnose der bösartigen Geschwülste [The microscopic diagnosis of malignant tumors.]. A. Hirschwald, Berlin
4. Bignold LP, Coghlan BLD, Jersmann HPA (2007) David Paul von Hansemann: contributions to oncology. Context, comments and translations. Birkhauser, Basel
5. Broders AC (1920) Squamous cell epithelioma of the lip: a study of five hundred thirty-seven cases. JAMA 74:656–664
6. Broders AC (1926) Carcinoma: grading and practical applications. Arch Pathol 2:376–381
7. Greenough RB (1925) Varying degrees of malignancy in cancer of the breast. J Cancer Res 9:425–463
8. Dukes CE (1937) Histologic grading of cancer. Proc R Soc Med 30:371–376
9. Henson DE (1988) The histological grading of neoplasms. Arch Pathol Lab Med 112:1091–1096
10. Collan Y (1989) General principles of grading lesions in diagnostic histopathology. Pathol Res Pract 185:539–543
11. Humphrey PA (2003) Prostate pathology. American Society of Clinical Pathology Press, Chicago, pp 339–340
12. Carriaga MT, Henson DE (1995) The histologic grading of cancer. Cancer 75:406–421
13. Haagensen CD (1933) The basis for histologic grading of carcinoma of the breast. Am J Cancer 1:285–327
14. Cross SS (1998) Grading and scoring in histopathology. Histopathology 33:99–106
15. Epstein JI, Allsbrook WC Jr, Amin MB et al (2005) The 2005 International Society of Urologic Pathology (ISUP) consensus conference on Gleason grading of prostatic carcinoma. Am J Surg Pathol 29:1228–1242
16. Egevad L, Allsbrook WC Jr, Epstein JI (2005) Current practice of Gleason grading among genitourinary pathologists. Hum Pathol 36:5–9
17. Meyer JS, Alvarez C, Milikowski C et al (2005) Breast carcinoma malignancy grading by bloom-Richardson vs proliferation index: reproducibility of grade and advantages of proliferation index. Mod Pathol 18:1067–1078
18. Kroger N, Milde-Langosch K, Riethdorf S et al (2006) Prognostic and predictive effects of immunohistochemical factors in high-risk primary breast cancer patients. Clin Cancer Res 12:159–168
19. Habuchi T, Marberger M, Droller MJ et al (2005) Prognostic markers for bladder cancer: international consensus panel on bladder tumor markers. Urology 66(Suppl 1):64–74
20. Scott IS, Morris LS, Rushbrook SM et al (2005) Immunohistochemical estimation of cell cycle entry and phase distribution in astrocytomas: applications in diagnostic neuropathology. Neuropathol Appl Neurobiol 31:455–466
21. Quinones-Hinojosa A, Sanai N, Smith JS, McDermott MW (2005) Techniques to assess the proliferative potential of brain tumors. J Neurooncol 74:19–30
22. Giordana MT, D'Agostino C, Pollo B et al (2005) Anaplasia is rare and does not influence prognosis in adult medulloblastoma. J Neuropathol Exp Neurol 64:869–874
23. Deyrup AT, Weiss SW (2006) Grading of soft tissue sarcomas: the challenge of providing precise information in an imprecise world. Histopathology 48:42–50
24. Dong F, Wang C, Farris AB et al (2012) Impact on the clinical outcome of prostate cancer by the 2005 International Society of Urological Pathology modified Gleason grading system. Am J Surg Pathol 36:838–843
25. Huttner A (2012) Overview of primary brain tumors: pathologic classification, epidemiology, molecular biology, and prognostic markers. Hematol Oncol Clin North Am 26:715–732
26. Rosai J (2011) Rosai and Ackerman's surgical pathology, 10th edn. Mosby/Elsevier, Edinburgh, pp 2513–2515

Nina Gale and Nina Zidar

2.1 Introduction

Head and neck tumors most often originate from the squamous epithelium, but they can also arise from the sinonasal mucosa and salivary glands. Squamous cell carcinoma (SCC) of this region is the sixth commonest cancer worldwide and thus forms a significant part of routine work in pathology. Benign and potentially malignant intraepithelial lesions, carcinoma in situ, and invasive SCC are by far the most frequent entities in this region. The grading of these lesions is of considerable clinical significance and is performed routinely. In addition to SCC and its variants, other, although infrequent, malignant tumors can be found in the head and neck region. Some of them are identical to homonymous tumors in other parts of the body, such as adenocarcinoma, malignant tumors of the salivary glands, and neuroendocrine carcinomas, whereas others, such as sinonasal undifferentiated carcinoma and olfactory neuroblastomas, are unique to this region. This chapter will review the most important malignant tumors and precursor lesions in this part of the body.

2.2 Squamous Intraepithelial Lesions of the Mouth and Larynx

It is widely accepted that the transition from a normal epithelium to SCC of the oral and laryngeal mucosa is a lengthy, comprehensive, and multistage process, causally related to a progressive accumulation of genetic changes leading to the selection of a clonal population of transformed epithelial cells. The entire spectrum of histological changes occurring in this process has recently been cumulatively designated squamous intraepithelial lesions (SILs), ranging from squamous hyperplasia to carcinoma in situ (CIS) [1, 2]. SILs of the oral and laryngeal mucosa are usually defined clinically as leukoplakia, erythroplakia (white or reddish plaques), and chronic laryngitis. Tobacco, whether smoked or chewed, and alcohol abuse, and especially a combination of these two detrimental factors, are major identifiable risk factors for oral and laryngeal SILs [1–5]. However, human papilloma virus (HPV) infection, with a high prevalence of HPV 16 and 18 genotypes, may also be implicated in oral leukoplakia as an infecting agent. HPV DNA prevalence of potentially malignant lesions in oral cavity ranges from 0 to 85 % [6, 7].

Regrettably, neither generally accepted criteria nor unified terminology has to date been provided for a histological grading system of oral and laryngeal SILs. Evidence of the inability to set up a single, unified classification of SILs was manifested in the World Health Organization

N. Gale, M.D. (✉) • N. Zidar, M.D.
Faculty of Medicine,
Institute of Pathology, University of Ljubljana,
Ljubljana, Slovenia
e-mail: nina.gale@mf.uni-lj.si

I. Damjanov, F. Fan (eds.), *Cancer Grading Manual*,
DOI 10.1007/978-3-642-34516-6_2, © Springer-Verlag Berlin Heidelberg 2013

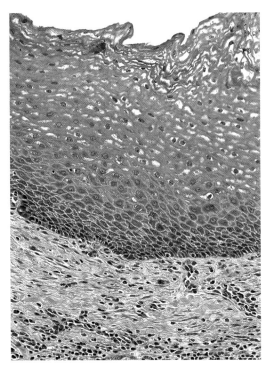

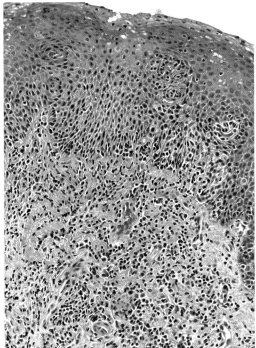

Fig. 2.1 Squamous cell hyperplasia. The prickle cell layer is thickened, but the basal layer is of normal thickness

Fig. 2.2 Basal and parabasal cell hyperplasia. The layers of basal and parabasal cells extend up to the middle of epithelial thickness; the upper part of the prickle cell layer shows no alterations

(WHO) classification of head and neck tumors, published in 2005, in which three different grading systems were presented: the dysplasia system, the classification of squamous intraepithelial neoplasia (SIN), and the classification which incorporates the tenets of the European consensus system known as the Ljubljana classification. The Ljubljana system nominally recognizes four grades and, from prognostic points of view, three groups: simple hyperplasia (SH) and basal/parabasal cell hyperplasia (BPH) are mainly benign categories with a minimum risk of malignant alteration, atypical hyperplasia (AH) or risky epithelium is potentially, and carcinoma in situ (CIS) actually a malignant lesion [1, 2].

- *Squamous Cell Hyperplasia.* This benign hyperplastic process shows thickening of the prickle cell layer. The basal and parabasal layers are unchanged (Fig. 2.1).
- *Basal and Parabasal Cell Hyperplasia.* In this lesion, there is an increased thickness of basal and parabasal cells in the lower half of

the epithelium; the upper part contains regular prickle cells. Stratification is preserved. Augmented basal and parabasal cells show moderately enlarged nuclei; rare regular mitoses may be seen in or near the basal layer (Fig. 2.2).

- *Atypical Hyperplasia or Risky Epithelium.* This potentially malignant lesion is characterized by the preserved stratification of squamous cells, which, however, show mild to moderate cytological atypia. The cells also have an increased nuclear to cytoplasmic ratio. Altered epithelial cells are mainly perpendicularly oriented to the basement membrane and occupy the lower half or more of the entire epithelium. Mitoses are increased in number and are found in the lower two-thirds of the epithelium. Mitoses are rarely, if ever, abnormal. Dyskeratotic cells are frequently present. Two subtypes are recognized: basal and spinous cell type (Fig. 2.3).

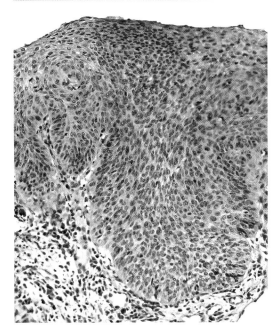

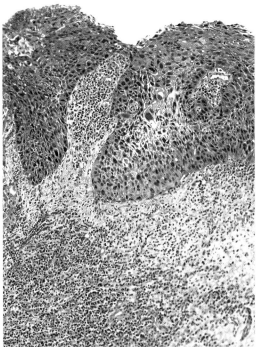

Fig. 2.3 Atypical hyperplasia. The basaloid cells, which show mild to moderate atypia but the stratification of cells is preserved, occupy the whole thickness of the epithelium. The cells also have an increased nuclear-cytoplasmic ratio

Fig. 2.4 Squamous cell carcinoma in situ. The epithelium shows a loss of normal stratification. The cells show moderate to severe atypias and increased mitotic activity

• *Carcinoma In Situ.* This lesion is characterized by a loss of epithelial stratification, moderate to severe cytological atypia of epithelial cells, and an increased number of mitotic figures within the whole epithelium, which are often abnormal. Two subtypes are found: basal and spinous cell type (Fig. 2.4).

2.2.1   Comments

1. Traditional light microscopic examination remains the most reliable method for determining an accurate diagnosis of SILs, in spite of certain subjectivity in interpretation.
2. The Ljubljana classification has been found to be precise for daily diagnostic work and provides data that have been shown to be closely correlated to the biological behavior of the lesions [1, 2]. The eventual outcome of laryngeal SILs patients so graded justifies the proposal for separating the lesions into a benign group (SH and BPH) and a potentially

malignant group (AH), showing malignant transformation in 0.9 and 11 % of cases, respectively [1]. Conversely, the results of malignant transformation studies vary considerably for each particular grade classified according to the dysplasia and squamous intraepithelial neoplasia (SIN) systems, as follows: squamous hyperplasia from 0 to 4.1 %, group of mild dysplasia and SIN I from 0 to 11 %, group of moderate dysplasia and SIN II from 4 to 24 %, and group of severe dysplasia and SIN III from 9.3 to 57 % [1].
3. Malignant transformation rates of oral leukoplakia range from 0.13 to 17.7 %. Leukoplakia of the tongue and floor of the mouth shows a higher risk of malignant transformation according to some authors, while others have not found specific oral subsets at high risk [6, 7]. Erythroplakia has the highest transformation rate among all precursor lesions, ranging from 14.3 to 50.0 % [8].

2.3 Squamous Cell Carcinoma of the Head and Neck

SCC is the most common malignant tumor of the head and neck accounting for approximately 90 % of all malignant tumors at this location. The majority are conventional-type SCC. The common locations include the oral cavity, oropharynx, hypopharynx, and the larynx. Less frequently it arises in other locations, such as the nasal cavity and paranasal sinuses and the nasopharynx.

SCC is traditionally graded into well differentiated (grade 1), moderately differentiated (grade 2), and poorly differentiated SCC (grade 3) according to the degree of differentiation, cellular pleomorphism, and mitotic activity. Although keratinization is more likely to be present in well- or moderately differentiated SCC, it should not be considered an important histological criterion in grading SCC [8].

- *Grade 1: Well-Differentiated Squamous Cell Carcinoma.* This tumor resembles closely normal squamous epithelium and contains varying proportions of large, differentiated keratinocyte-like squamous cells and small basal-type cells, which are usually located at the periphery of the tumor islands. Intercellular bridges are always present. Keratin pearls are frequently found; mitoses are scanty (Fig. 2.5a).
- *Grade 2: Moderately Differentiated Squamous Cell Carcinoma.* This tumor exhibits more nuclear pleomorphism and an increased number of mitoses, including abnormal mitoses; there is usually less keratinization (Fig. 2.5b).
- *Grade 3: Poorly Differentiated Squamous Cell Carcinoma.* In this tumor, basal-type cells predominate, with a high mitotic rate, including abnormal mitoses, barely discernible intercellular bridges, and minimal, if any, keratinization (Fig. 2.5c).

Several variants of SCC have been described, including verrucous carcinoma, spindle cell carcinoma, basaloid SCC, papillary SCC, lymphoepithelial carcinoma, adenoid (acantholytic) SCC, and adenosquamous carcinoma. Their recognition is important because most of them are true clinicopathologic entities, with a different prognostic implication: basaloid SCC, adenosquamous carcinoma, and lymphoepithelial carcinoma are more aggressive than conventional SCC, while verrucous SCC and, arguably, papillary SCC have a better prognosis than conventional SCC [7].

SCC of the head and neck has been traditionally etiologically related to tobacco smoking or chewing and alcohol abuse. Recent studies have discovered a new etiologic agent – infection with HPV, particularly HPV types 16 and 18. These tumors show rather characteristic clinicopathologic features and mostly arise in the oropharynx (palatinal and lingual tonsils). HPV infection in SCC at other sites is exceptional [9–11]. Morphologically, HPV-positive SCCs are usually similar to the basaloid SCC and occasionally to papillary or lymphoepithelial SCCs, whereas the role of HPV in some other SCC subtypes (e.g., verrucous carcinoma) is controversial. Spindle cell carcinoma and acantholytic SCC are probably not HPV-related variants of SCC.

Most HPV-positive SCCs lack keratinization, and some authors have proposed the term "non-keratinizing HPV-positive SCC." They are usually composed of tumor cells of basaloid appearance, which lack maturation, exhibiting at least moderate degree of atypia (Fig. 2.6a). Despite its resemblance to basaloid SCC, its behavior and prognosis is different, and determining HPV status has an important prognostic implication. HPV-positive SCC has been demonstrated to respond well to radiotherapy and to have an improved survival in comparison to HPV-negative SCC [9–12]. It has been therefore proposed that HPV status should be assessed in all cases of basaloid SCC, particularly of the oropharynx. At the present time, in situ hybridization (Fig. 2.6c) and polymerase chain reaction (PCR) are the most reliable methods for determining HPV status [11].

HPV-positive SCCs overexpress the p16 gene product (Fig. 2.6b). It has been hypothesized that this effect is a consequence of the distinct molecular mechanisms of carcinogenesis associated with HPV infection through pRb inactivation by the HPV E7 oncoprotein and upregulation of the p16 protein [12].

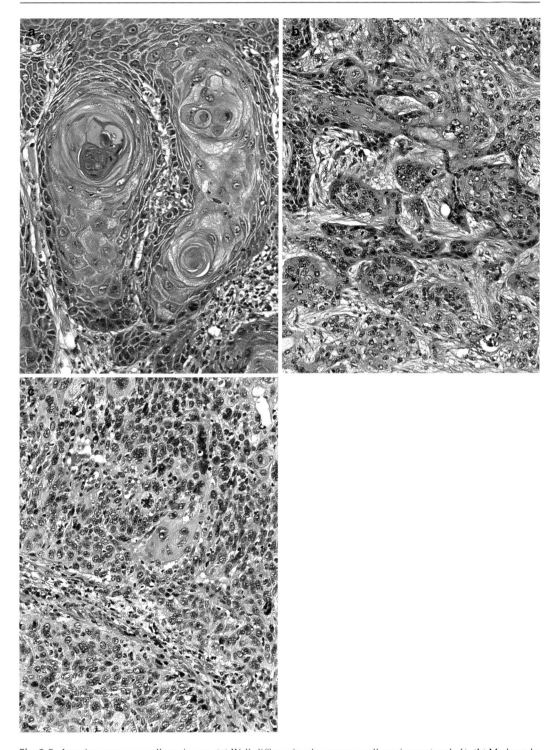

Fig. 2.5 Invasive squamous cell carcinoma. (**a**) Well-differentiated squamous cell carcinoma (grade 1). (**b**) Moderately differentiated squamous cell carcinoma (grade 2). (**c**) Poorly differentiated squamous cell carcinoma (grade 3)

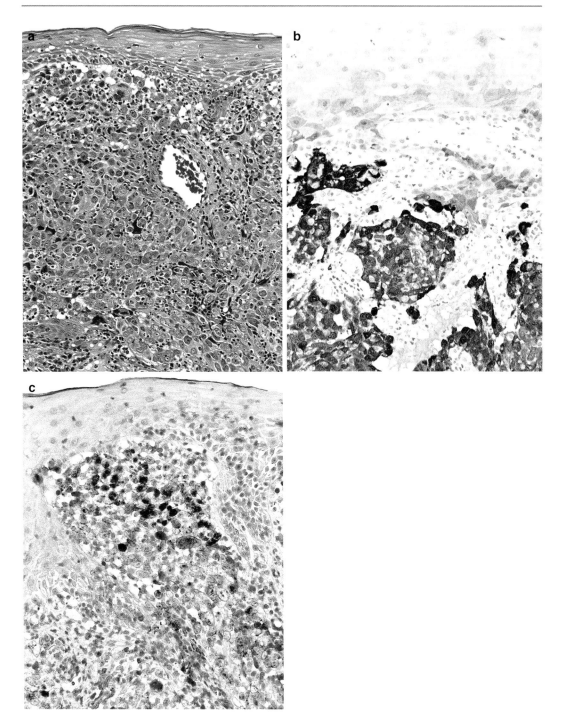

Fig. 2.6 Non-keratinizing squamous cell carcinoma of the palatinal tonsil. (**a**) The tumor is composed of nests of cells showing no signs of keratinization. (**b**) Immunohistochemistry shows diffuse strong expression of p16. (**c**) In situ hybridization reveals HPV type 16/18 in the majority of tumor cells

Overexpression of p16 is generally accepted as a surrogate marker of HPV infection, though lacking the sufficient specificity to replace in situ hybridization or PCR. The general consensus is that p16 immunohistochemistry and HPV in situ hybridization are complementary, with p16 being an appropriate screening tool [11].

2.3.1   Comments

1. Traditional grading of SCC is subjective, and its prognostic significance is controversial. Some studies have suggested that the grade of SCC has a significant influence on prognosis [13, 14], while others have not confirmed this observation [15].
2. Variations in differentiation are frequently observed within a single tumor, but grading must be based on the worst differentiated area.
3. A subset of SCCs in the head and neck are associated to HPV infection, particularly in the oropharynx. These are usually non-keratinizing tumors with basaloid appearance. Determining HPV status is important because HPV-positive SCCs are more radiosensitive and have a better prognosis than HPV-negative SCCs.

2.4   Nasopharyngeal Carcinoma

Nasopharyngeal carcinoma (NPC) arises from the nasopharyngeal epithelium and shows squamous cell differentiation. The 2005 WHO classification recognizes three main groups of these tumors: keratinizing NPC, non-keratinizing (differentiated and undifferentiated) NPC, and basaloid NPC [16, 17]. Etiologically, NPC is related to race, Epstein-Barr virus (EBV) infection (non-keratinizing NPC), and genetic changes. NPC is a rare tumor, with fewer than 1/100,000/year, except in regions of South China, North Africa, and the Arctic region (20–30/100,000/year). The lateral and posterior-superior walls of the nasopharynx are the commonest locations of the tumors, which are intimately related to the nasopharyngeal lymphoid tissue. Clinically, a considerable number of patients may have occult primary tumors, and the first presentation is cervical lymph node metastases localized in the posterior cervical triangle or superior jugular region. Although a multistep evolution of NPC is proposed, precursor lesions and carcinoma in situ have been identified in only 3–8 % of cases. The 5-year disease-specific survival is 81 % and overall survival about 75 %.

- *Keratinizing, Conventional Squamous Cell Carcinoma*. This type of NPC accounts for about 25 % of cases and microscopically shows definite evidence of squamous differentiation (keratin pearls and intercellular bridges). Just as other squamous cell carcinomas, they are graded into well-differentiated, moderately, or poorly differentiated neoplasms. It is not usually related to EBV infection.

- *Non-keratinizing NPC, Differentiated and Undifferentiated Carcinoma*. This is the commonest form of NPC, accounting for about 75 % cases. Subclassification into differentiated and undifferentiated subtypes is clinically not decisive; both subtypes are related to EBV infection in 75–100 % of cases. The differentiated type is composed of solid sheets and interconnecting cords of focally stratified neoplastic hyperchromatic cells of medium size with evident nuclear pleomorphism, increased mitotic activity, and increased nuclear-cytoplasmic ratio. There is no evidence of keratinization (Fig. 2.7). The undifferentiated type is characterized by well-defined epithelial aggregates or a syncytial growth pattern, also called the "Regaud type," or by ill-defined sheets, clusters, or dissociated cells, intermingled with lymphocytes, also called the "Schmincke type." Syncytial-appearing cells have an indistinct cell membrane and large, round to oval vesicular nuclei with prominent eosinophilic nucleoli. Tumor cells have scant, usually amphophilic cytoplasm. These cells are larger than cells of the differentiated type of NPC. Stromal lymphocytes are part of the native lymphoid tissue of the nasopharyngeal mucosa (Fig. 2.8). Overlapping of differentiated and undifferentiated types of

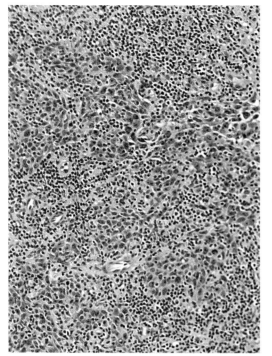

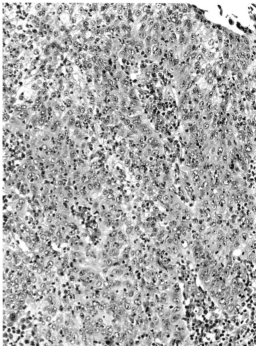

Fig. 2.7 Non-keratinizing differentiated nasopharyngeal carcinoma. Interconnecting cords of moderately pleomorphic cell with hyperchromatic nuclei infiltrated and surrounded by abundant nonneoplastic lymphocytes

Fig. 2.8 Non-keratinizing undifferentiated nasopharyngeal carcinoma. Cohesive islands and trabeculae of large cells with round vesicular nuclei and prominent eosinophilic nucleoli infiltrated by lymphocytes

non-keratinizing NPC may be present. Precise separation is difficult to achieve and has no clinical and prognostic significance [16, 17]. NPC is classified according to its dominant component.

2.4.1 Comments

Non-keratinizing NPC has a broad differential diagnosis including malignant melanoma, lymphoma, olfactory neuroblastoma, neuroendocrine carcinoma, Ewing sarcoma, and undifferentiated sinonasal carcinoma (SNUC). A wide spectrum of immunohistochemical markers and in situ hybridization for EBV detection has to be applied. Non-keratinizing NPC shows characteristic positivity for cytokeratins CK5/6 and CK13 and EBV. Poor prognosis is associated with advanced clinical stage, cranial nerves involvement, keratinizing histology, and absence of EBV [16].

2.5 Sinonasal Carcinomas

Sinonasal malignant tumors are rare, representing about 0.2–0.8 % of all human malignant neoplasms and about 3 % of all malignancies of the head and neck. They mostly originate in the maxillary sinus (60 %), followed by the nasal cavity (20–30 %), ethmoid sinus (10–15 %), and the frontal and sphenoid sinus (1 %). The incidence of these tumors is very low in most populations, except in the East and Southeast Asia. Squamous cell carcinoma is the most common form of sinonasal carcinomas. Poorly differentiated neoplasms predominate over well-differentiated ones within this area.

2.5.1 Squamous Cell Carcinoma

The 2005 WHO classification of head and neck tumors proposed the following histopathological classification of sinonasal SCC: keratinizing SCC, non-keratinizing (cylindrical cell or transitional) carcinoma, and variants of SCC. These tumors show a wide range of differentiation, and particularly poorly differentiated forms may show a considerable overlap histologically, making their distinction difficult, especially in small biopsies [17, 18]. However, compared to conventional SCC, the non-keratinizing type is above all a locally aggressive tumor and mainly has a better prognosis than the conventional, keratinizing form. Only non-keratinizing carcinoma is a distinctive phenotype of the sinonasal tract, while keratinizing SCC and its variants are identical to homonymous tumors in the head and neck region and other parts of the human body.

- *Non-keratinizing Carcinoma.* This distinctive form of SCC, derived from the respiratory (Schneiderian) epithelium, is composed of thick ribbons of multilayered cylindrical cells, often surrounded by the basement membrane. Inverted growth arising from the surface epithelium in the form of interconnected bands of neoplastic epithelium is the characteristic hallmark of this type of sinonasal carcinoma. The elongated or oval cells show nuclear pleomorphism, hyperchromasia, and increased mitotic activity. The cells arranged along the basement membrane may be perpendicularly oriented (Fig. 2.9).

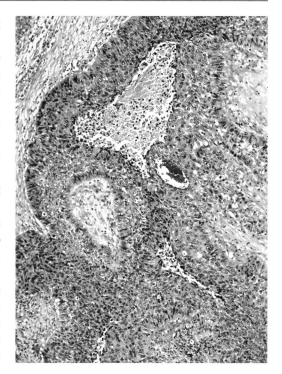

Fig. 2.9 Non-keratinizing sinonasal squamous cell carcinoma. Thick ribbons of polystratified cylindrical and basal cells, form palisade arrangements, oriented perpendicularly to the basement membrane

2.5.2 Sinonasal Undifferentiated Carcinoma (SNUC)

This high-grade neoplasm is very rare, characterized as a highly aggressive and clinicopathologically distinctive cancer of uncertain histogenesis with extremely poor prognosis. Microscopically, it is composed of medium- to large-sized undifferentiated cells, which form nests, sheets, and ribbons with frequent areas of central necrosis and a tendency to perineural and intravascular invasion. The cells have round to oval large hyperchromatic to vesicular nuclei; nucleoli are typically prominent but in some cases may also be inconspicuous. Most cells have a small amount of cytoplasm with poorly defined cell membranes. However, distinct cell borders are also described in some cases. A nuclear-cytoplasmic ratio is high. Increased mitotic activity is evident, as are atypical mitoses as well as numerous apoptotic cells (Fig. 2.10). There is no evidence of squamous or glandular differentiation; neurofibrillary material and true neural rosettes have also not been identified [19, 20].

2.5.3 Adenocarcinomas

These neoplasms of the sinonasal tract are classified into salivary and non-salivary types. The first group includes salivary-specific tumors, such as mucoepidermoid carcinoma and adenoid cystic carcinoma. The non-salivary group is divided into intestinal and non-intestinal types. The latter are further divided into low- and high-grade tumors. All adenocarcinomas of the sinonasal area together, including salivary gland-type malignant tumors, comprise 10–20 % of primary sinonasal malignant neoplasms.

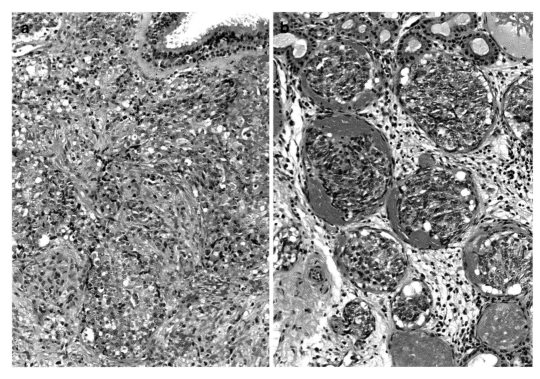

Fig. 2.10 Sinonasal undifferentiated carcinoma. (**a**) Irregular cords and islands of medium-sized, undifferentiated cells with slightly hyperchromatic nuclei and incon- spicuous nucleoli surrounded by amphophilic cytoplasm. (**b**) Intravascular invasion is a frequent finding in SNUC

• *Intestinal-Type Adenocarcinomas.* The 2005 WHO classification of head and neck tumors accepted both the Barnes [21] and Kleinsasser and Schroeder [22] classifications of intestinal-type adenocarcinomas (Table 2.1). The two classifications share many similarities, and their use depends on personal preference. The papillary type (well-differentiated, papillary tubular cylinder cell I or PTCC I) displays a predominant papillary growth pattern with occasional tubular glands, cellular atypias are minimal, and mitotic activity is low. Columnar cells are frequently arranged with the long axis perpendicular to the basement membrane; they may also be stratified. The cells have eosinophilic cytoplasm and round to oval vesicular or hyperchromatic nuclei. Focally goblet cells may also be present (Fig. 2.11). Some neoplasms are only in situ, but most of them are obviously invasive. The colonic type (PTCC II) resembles large intestine cancers, with moderately differentiated glands. A papillary pattern

Table 2.1 Histological classification of sinonasal intestinal-type adenocarcinomas

Barnes [21]	Kleinsasser and Schroeder [22]
Papillary type	PTCC I
Colonic type	PTCC II
Solid type	PTCC III
Mucinous type	Alveolar goblet cell
	Signet-ring cell
Mixed	Transitional cell

Source: Modified from Barnes [21] and Kleinsasser and Schoeder [22]
PTCC papillary, tubular, cylindrical cell

is infrequent; stratified cells show more pronounced atypias and mitoses (Fig. 2.12). This type is the most frequent among all intestinal-type adenocarcinomas. The solid variant (PTCC III) shows a diffuse proliferation of smaller cuboidal cells with pronounced cellular atypias (Fig. 2.13). Mitoses, also atypical, are numerous. Neoplasms with the production of mucin

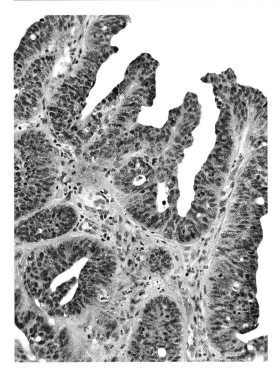

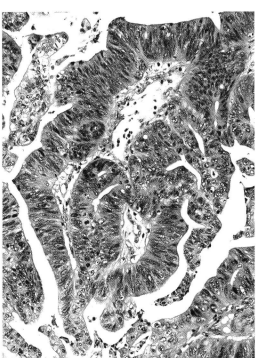

Fig. 2.11 Intestinal-type adenocarcinoma, papillary type. Papillary outgrowth of the pseudostratified epithelial cells and tubuloglandular formations resemble primary intestinal adenocarcinoma

Fig. 2.12 Intestinal-type adenocarcinoma, colonic type. The tumor has a tubuloglandular growth pattern and form a few papillae, thus resembling colonic adenocarcinoma

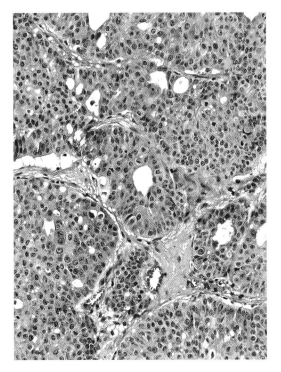

(alveolar goblet signet ring) are divided into two types. One type is characterized by a solid island of cells, short papillary fronds and glands, as well as proliferations of signet-ring cells lying in the mucomyxoid stroma. Mucin is predominantly intracellular. The other type is composed of distended glands with abundant mucin production and surrounded by one layer of cylindrical or goblet cells. Pools of mucinous substance are also evident around glandular structures, often separated by thin strands of fibrous stroma, creating an alveolar-like pattern (Fig. 2.14). A mixed (transitional) pattern is composed of two or more of the previously described types [23, 24].

- *Non-intestinal-Type Adenocarcinomas.* These tumors are neither intestinal nor salivary gland

Fig. 2.13 Intestinal-type adenocarcinoma, partially solid type. Parts of the tumor are solid, whereas others consist of tubules

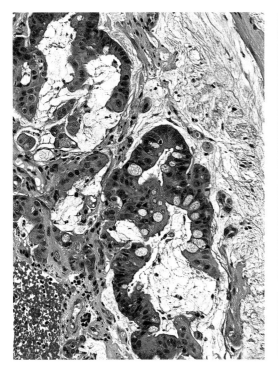

Fig. 2.14 Intestinal-type adenocarcinoma, mucinous type. Abundant extracellular mucin forms pools containing scattered glands and numerous goblet cells

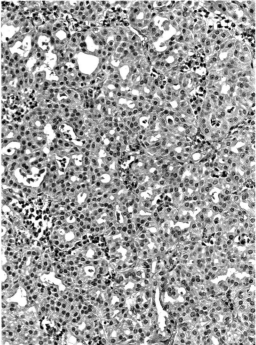

Fig. 2.15 Non-intestinal-type adenocarcinoma, low grade. Tumor is composed of glands in a back-to-back pattern. These neoplastic glands are lined by a single layer of cuboidal cells, which lack cellular and nuclear atypia

adenocarcinomas. They are divided into low- and high-grade neoplasms. Low-grade tumors are composed of infiltrative small uniform glands with a back-to-back pattern without intermingled fibrous stroma; some irregular cystic spaces may be present. Glands are lined by uniform cuboidal to columnar cells with uniform round nuclei. Cellular and nuclear pleomorphism is mild; mitoses are infrequent (Fig. 2.15). Rare variants include papillary, oncocytic, or clear cell patterns of adenocarcinomas. The high-grade variant shows a predominantly solid- or sheetlike growth, and a papillary or glandular pattern may also be present. Tumor cell are pleomorphic, with increased mitotic activity; necroses and perineural growth are frequently present (Fig. 2.16).

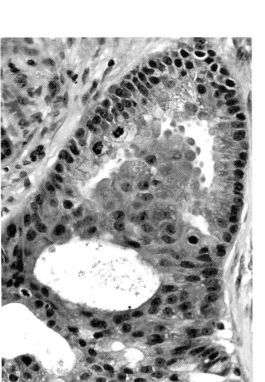

Fig. 2.16 Non-intestinal-type adenocarcinoma, high grade. Glandular growth pattern, exhibiting increased cellular and nuclear atypias and increased mitotic activity

2.5.4 Comments

1. SNUC must be immunohistochemically distinguished from other round cell tumors of this area, such as olfactory neuroblastoma, neuroendocrine carcinoma, peripheral neuroectodermal tumor/Ewing sarcoma, rhabdomyosarcoma, and malignant lymphoma. It is characteristically positive only for keratin; other markers, especially endocrine, are exceptionally positive.

2. The histologic subtypes and grading of intestinal types of adenocarcinomas are important predictive factors for local recurrence, metastatic spread, and survival. The papillary type (PTCC I) has an indolent course, and 5-year survival is about 80 %; conversely, the solid type (PTCC III) and mucinous type have very poor survival rates [22].

3. The prognosis for non-intestinal-type adenocarcinomas strongly correlates with their grades [23]. Low-grade tumors have an excellent prognosis, while the 3-year survival of patients with high-grade neoplasms is only about 20 % (Barnes et al. 2005).

2.6 Neuroendocrine Carcinoma

Neuroendocrine carcinomas (NECs) of the head and neck are uncommon. Their classification and grading have been recently the subject of debate, mostly due to reluctance to abandon old terminology (carcinoid, atypical carcinoid) instead of the newly proposed term "neuroendocrine carcinoma." In the WHO classification, both the old and the new terminologies are included.

Similarly to other locations, NEC of the head and neck are divided into well-differentiated NEC (carcinoid), moderately differentiated NEC (atypical carcinoid), and poorly differentiated NEC (small cell carcinoma). The most common locations in the head and neck region are the larynx [25], pharynx, and salivary glands. They are identified by immunohistochemistry showing expression of neuroendocrine markers, such as synaptophysin, chromogranin, Leu-7, CD56, CD57, and neurofilament protein. NEC may be associated with a paraneoplastic syndrome.

- *Well-Differentiated Neuroendocrine Carcinoma (Carcinoid)*
  Well-differentiated NEC is the least common type of head and neck NEC. Microscopically, it is composed of small uniform cell growing in islands, ribbons, and cords, occasionally forming gland-like structures. The nuclei are round, with finely dispersed chromatin and inconspicuous nucleoli; the cytoplasm is scant, clear, or eosinophilic. Mitoses are sparse or absent, and there is no necrosis or cellular pleomorphism.
  The treatment of choice is complete but conservative surgical excision. Neck dissection is not indicated. Radiotherapy and chemotherapy have not proven effective. Prognosis is favorable, though metastases to the lymph nodes, liver, bones, and skin have been reported in one-third of patients.

- *Moderately Differentiated Neuroendocrine Carcinoma (Atypical Carcinoid)*
  It is the most frequent type of NEC in the larynx constituting 54 % of all laryngeal NEC. Microscopically, the tumor grows in rounded nests, trabeculae, cords, ribbons, and glandular structures; the tumor cells are round, with round nuclei and moderate amount of cytoplasm which is slightly eosinophilic or occasionally oncocytic. In contrast to well-differentiated NEC, cellular pleomorphism, increased mitotic activity, and necroses are frequently present in moderately differentiated NEC. Vascular and perineural invasion may be present (Fig. 2.17).
  Differential diagnosis includes paraganglioma, adenocarcinoma, other neuroendocrine carcinomas, and medullary carcinoma of the thyroid gland.
  Moderately differentiated NEC is an aggressive, potentially lethal tumor. Lymph node metastases have been reported in 43 % of patients, cutaneous metastases in 22 %, and distant metastases in 44 % of patients, mostly to the lungs, liver, and bones. Surgery is the treatment of choice. Neck dissection is also advised because of the high incidence of

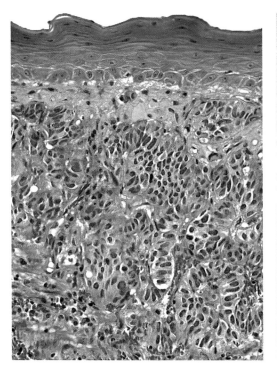 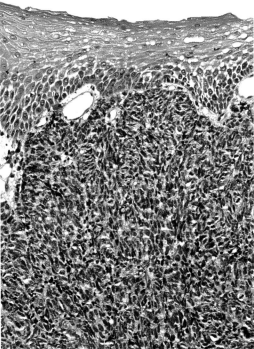

Fig. 2.17 Moderately differentiated neuroendocrine carcinoma (atypical carcinoid). The tumor grows in rounded nests; the tumor cells are ovoid with elongated nuclei and moderate amount of cytoplasm which is slightly eosinophilic

Fig. 2.18 Poorly differentiated neuroendocrine carcinoma (small cell carcinoma). It is composed of closely packed small cells with hyperchromatic and spindle nuclei and very scant cytoplasm. Necrosis and mitoses are frequently present

cervical lymph node metastases. Radiation and chemotherapy have not been effective. The 5- and 10-year survival rates are 48 and 30 %, respectively [7].

- *Poorly Differentiated Neuroendocrine Carcinoma (Small Cell Carcinoma)*
  Poorly differentiated NEC is the least differentiated and the most aggressive type of NEC. It is rare, accounting for less than 0.5 % of all laryngeal carcinomas. Microscopically, it is identical to their pulmonary counterparts. It is composed of closely packed small cells with hyperchromatic round, oval, or spindle nuclei and very scant cytoplasm. Necroses, mitoses, as well as vascular and perineural invasion are frequently present (Fig. 2.18). Few cases of head and neck NECs have been described, consisting of large cells with more cytoplasm, resembling large cell NEC in the lungs and other locations [26]. In the differential diagnosis, the possibility of a metastasis from the lung must be excluded.

Poorly differentiated NEC must also not be confused with the basaloid squamous carcinoma, malignant lymphoma, and malignant melanoma.

The clinical course is aggressive, characterized by early metastases to the regional lymph nodes and distant sites, especially to the lungs, bones, and liver. Radiation with chemotherapy is the treatment of choice. Surgical therapy is not indicated because most patients have disseminated disease at presentation. Prognosis is poor; the 2- and 5-year survival rates are 16 and 5 %, respectively [7].

2.7 Olfactory Neuroblastoma

Olfactory neuroblastoma (ON) is a rare malignant neuroectodermal tumor arising from the olfactory membrane and represents 2–3 % of tumors of the sinonasal tract [27]. ON arises from the olfactory

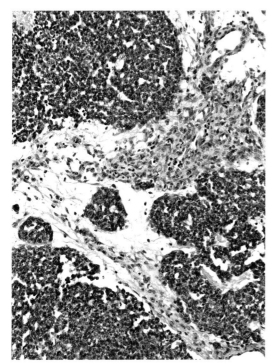

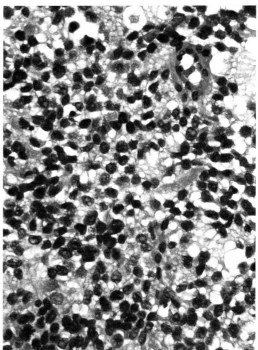

Fig. 2.19 Olfactory neuroblastoma, grade I. Well-defined lobular growth of "small round blue cells" is characteristic of a low-grade tumor

Fig. 2.20 Olfactory neuroblastoma, grade II. Small cells hyperchromatic nuclei without conspicuous cellular variability are embedded in neurofibrillar matrix

neuroepithelium, which normally covers the superior third of the nasal septum, cribriform plate, and superior turbinate. Rarely, it arises in the paranasal sinuses. ON has a bimodal age distribution, with peaks in the second and sixth decades. It often appears as a large, unilateral polypoid mass.

The microscopic appearance of ON depends on the degree of differentiation. A lobular pattern is almost always present, regardless of the tumor grade. ON characteristically consists of small, round, so-called blue cells, slightly larger than mature lymphocytes (Fig. 2.19). Nuclei are hyperchromatic, with regularly dispersed chromatin; nucleoli, if present, are inconspicuous. The cytoplasm is sparse. Cells, arranged in a syncytium, are nested in neurofibrillary processes (Fig. 2.20). The presence of cellular and nuclear pleomorphism and the number of mitoses and necroses depend on the tumor grade. ON are graded according to the criteria proposed by V. J. Hyams (Table 2.2). In grades I and II, they are absent or limited, but they are present in high-

grade tumors (III and IV). ON may show two types of rosettes: in the Homer-Wright pseudorosette, the tumor cells surround a central space filled with a finely fibrillar neural matrix; they are mainly seen in grades I and II. In Flexner-Wintersteiner true rosettes, the columnar tumor cells create a duct-like avascular space (Fig. 2.21); they may be present in grades III and IV. The lobules of tumor cells are surrounded by sustentacular cells, typically positive for S-100. ON has highly vascular and edematous stroma; calcifications may be present.

2.7.1   Comments

Immunohistochemistry is decisive for the diagnosis of ON, since the tumors are positive for neuroendocrine markers, while keratin is usually negative [20, 27]. Frequent local recurrences considerably influence the prognosis. Low-grade tumors have a reported 80 % 5-year survival

Table 2.2 Hyams grading system for olfactory neuroblastoma

Microscopic features	Grade I	Grade II	Grade III	Grade IV
Lobular pattern	++	++	+/−	−/+
Uniform nuclei	++	+/−	−/+	−
Mitoses	−	+	++	++
Calcification	+/−	+/−	−	−
Necrosis	−	−	+/−	++
Neurofibrillary background	+++	++	+/−	−
Homer-Wright rosettes	+/−	+/−	−	−
Flexner-Wintersteiner rosettes	−	−	++	−

Source: Modified from Hyams et al. (1988)

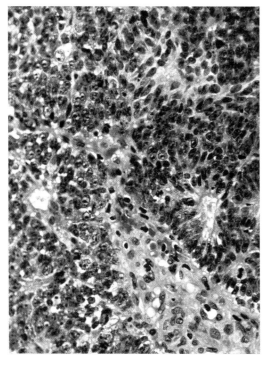

Fig. 2.21 Olfactory neuroblastoma, grade III. Lobules are formed of columnar cells with round, pale nuclei and eosinophilic nucleoli. Neoplastic cells create duct-like structures known as Flexner-Wintersteiner true rosettes

compared to 40 % 5-year survival for high-grade tumors [27].

2.8   Salivary Gland Carcinomas

Salivary gland carcinomas represent 3–5 % of all malignant tumors of the head and neck. The tumor type and histologic grade are important predictors of outcome. Low- and intermediate-grade carcinomas have a 5-year survival rate of 85–90 %, while high-grade carcinomas have a 5-year survival rate of roughly 40 % [28].

Nevertheless, all salivary gland carcinomas are not graded. Some of them are by definition high-grade tumors (e.g., salivary duct carcinoma, myoepithelial carcinoma, SCC), and others are low-grade tumors (e.g., polymorphous low-grade adenocarcinoma, acinic cell carcinoma, basal cell adenocarcinoma, epithelial-myoepithelial carcinoma). Very rarely low-grade tumors undergo high-grade transformation ("dedifferentiation"), becoming highly aggressive tumors that have a poor prognosis (e.g., acinic cell carcinoma, adenoid cystic carcinoma).

Two salivary gland carcinomas that are consistently graded are mucoepidermoid and adenoid cystic carcinoma. In addition, carcinoma ex pleomorphic adenoma must not be regarded as a specific diagnosis but a category in which the carcinoma should be typed, graded, and quantitated [28].

2.8.1   Mucoepidermoid Carcinoma

Mucoepidermoid carcinoma (MEC) is the most common malignant tumor of the salivary glands accounting for approximately 30 % of all malignant salivary gland tumors. In some patients, there is a history of exposure to ionizing radiation. Approximately 60 % of MECs arise in the major salivary glands (in the parotid gland and less frequently in the submandibular and very rarely in sublingual glands). The rest arise in the minor salivary glands, e.g., in the palate and

Table 2.3 The AFIP grading system for mucoepidermoid carcinomas

Histologic features	Point value
Intracystic component less than 20 %	2
Neural invasion	2
Necrosis	3
Mitoses (4 or more per 10 HPF)	3
Anaplasia	4

Modified from Luna [30]
Low grade: 0–4 points
Intermediate grade: 5–6 points
High grade: 7–14 points
AFIP Armed Forces Institute of Pathology, *HPF* high power field

Table 2.4 The Brandwein grading system for mucoepidermoid carcinomas

Histologic features	Point value
Intracystic component less than 25 %	2
Tumor invasion in form of small nests and islands	2
Pronounced nuclear atypia	2
Lymphovascular invasion	3
Invasion of bone	3
Perineural spread	3
Necrosis	3

Modified from Brandwein et al. [29]
Grade I: 0 points
Grade II: 2–3 points
Grade III: 4 or more points

buccal mucosa, tongue, gingiva, nasal cavity, larynx, and pharynx. Few cases have been described in the mandibula and maxilla (central MEC). MEC occurs at all ages, even in childhood, but it usually presents in the sixth and seventh decades, predominantly in males.

Microscopically, MEC is composed of varying proportion of mucinous, intermediate, squamous, and clear cells. On the basis of morphologic and cytologic features, MECs are classified as low-, intermediate-, and high-grade tumors. The suggested criteria for grading include the relative proportion of cell types, the proportion of tumor containing cysts, degree and pattern of invasion, mitotic rate, presence of vascular and perineural invasion, necrosis, and degree of nuclear and cellular atypias.

Several grading systems have been proposed, but none have been universally accepted. The most commonly used are the AFIP system and the Brandwein system [28–30] (Table 2.3). Comparing the two systems, it has been found that both are easy to reproduce and that the AFIP system tends to downgrade MEC in comparison to the Brandwein system [30] (Table 2.4).

- *Low-grade (grade I) MECs* usually have numerous cystic spaces, formed by various cell types and rare mitoses, and no perineural or vascular invasion are present. The tumor is typically well circumscribed, with expansive growth pattern at the invasive front (Fig. 2.22).
- *Intermediate-grade (grade II) MECs* usually have cysts occupying less than 20 % of the tumor, exhibit slight to moderate cellular

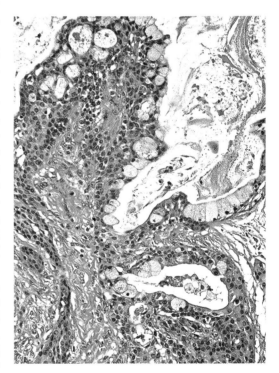

Fig. 2.22 Mucoepidermoid carcinoma, low grade, grade I. This cystic tumor is composed of numerous goblet and intermediate cells

polymorphism, and perineural invasion is often present. Unlike low-grade MEC, intermediate MEC usually has infiltrative pattern of growth at the invasive front (Fig. 2.23).

- *High-grade (grade III) MECs* are solid, anaplastic tumors with more than 4 mitoses per high power field, with scanty mucin production,

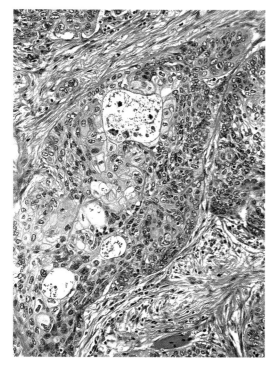

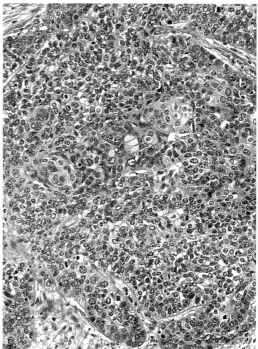

Fig. 2.23 Mucoepidermoid carcinoma, intermediate grade, grade II. This cystic tumor contains goblet, intermediate, and squamous cells, with only a few mitoses

Fig. 2.24 Mucoepidermoid carcinoma, high grade, grade III. This solid tumor is composed of moderately pleomorphic squamous cells with high mitotic rate and few goblet cells

and infiltrative growth pattern at the invasive front. Necroses and perineural and lymphovascular invasion are usually present (Fig. 2.24).

The behavior of MECs is related to the grade and stage of the disease, with the exception of submandibular MEC in which the behavior is unpredictable and correlates poorly with the grade and stage. The 5-year survival rate for MEC ranges from 92 to 100 % for low-grade MEC, 62 to 92 % for intermediate-grade MEC, and 0 to 43 % for high-grade MEC [28]. The best treatment is complete surgical excision. Radiotherapy has been reported to be successful in a limited number of patients. Neck dissection may be necessary, as 50 % of patients with MEC have metastases in the regional lymph nodes.

2.8.2 Adenoid Cystic Carcinoma

Adenoid cystic carcinoma (ACC) is a biphasic tumor composed of ductal and myoepithelial

cells. It is characterized by a slow but relentless progression, with local recurrences, late metastases, and usually a fatal outcome. It accounts for approximately 10 % of salivary gland tumors, arising most frequently in the parotid, submandibular, and minor salivary glands (in the palate, tongue, buccal mucosa, lip, floor of the mouth). ACC occurs in all age groups, with highest frequency in middle ages and older patients, with no apparent sex predilection.

Microscopically, ACC is characterized by histologically polymorphous but cytologically relatively uniform features. It consists of ductal and modified myoepithelial cells, with characteristically hyperchromatic, angular nuclei, and scant cytoplasm. ACC can exhibit three different growth patterns: tubular, solid, and cribriform. All three patterns may be present within the same tumor. In the tubular pattern (Fig. 2.25), ducts and tubules with central lumina are formed, lined by inner epithelial and outer myoepithelial cells. In the cribriform pattern (Swiss cheese-like pattern)

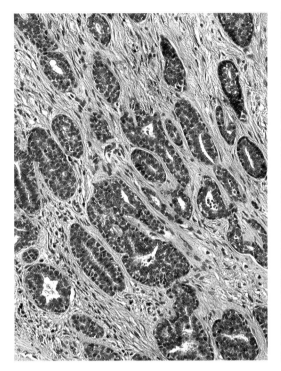

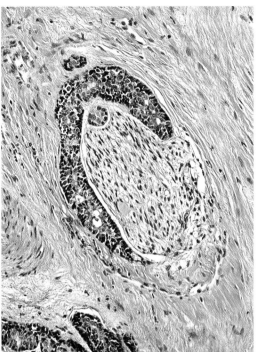

Fig. 2.25 Adenoid cystic carcinoma. The tumor has a tubular growth pattern

Fig 2.27 Adenoid cystic carcinoma. The tumor cells show perineural invasion

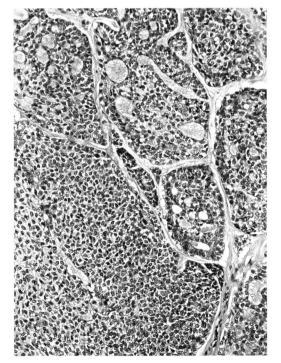

Fig. 2.26 Adenoid cystic carcinoma. The tumor displays two growth patterns, i.e., a cribriform and a solid growth pattern

(Fig. 2.26), tumor cells form nests with microcystic spaces, which are filled with hyaline or basophilic mucoid material. In the solid pattern, tumor cells grow in sheets (Fig. 2.26), lacking tubular and microcystic formation. The stroma in ACC is hyalinized and may exhibit mucinous or myxoid features. Perineural (Fig. 2.27) and intraneural invasion is commonly present. It is a characteristic, though not a pathognomonic feature of ACC, enabling tumor cells to extend far beyond the clinically apparent boundaries of the tumor [31].

ACC is usually graded according to the predominant growth pattern. Grade I tumors have a predominant tubular growth, grade II tumors are cribriform, and grade III have a solid growth pattern. Generally, ACC can be considered grade III if more than 30 % of the tumor shows a solid growth pattern, but some authors define the cutoff point at 50 %. Grading ACC has been shown to be prognostically important [28]. Tumor exhibiting cribriform and tubular patterns pursues a less aggressive course than those with a greater than 30 % of a solid component.

Regardless of the grade, ACCs are usually treated with surgery plus irradiation. The risk for lymph node metastases is low, and therefore neck dissection is not indicated in cases with clinically negative nodes. Some authors believe that neck dissection should only be performed in high-risk ACCs, e.g., in grade III tumors, and in ACC with transformation to high-grade tumors. The course of the disease is slow but relentless; the 5-year survival is 75–80 %, but 15-year survival is about 35 % [28].

2.8.3 Carcinoma ex Pleomorphic Adenoma

Carcinoma ex pleomorphic adenoma (CPA) is a malignant epithelial tumor arising in or from pleomorphic adenoma. These are rare tumors accounting for approx. 12 % of all salivary gland malignant tumors. They usually present at older age, in the sixth and seventh decade, about 10 years later than pleomorphic adenoma. They most commonly arise in the parotid gland, followed by the submandibular gland and minor salivary glands.

Microscopically, the proportion of the pleomorphic adenoma component varies from one tumor to another. It can be inconspicuous, and if suspected, extensive sampling may be necessary to find it. If not found, the diagnosis of CPA can only be made if there is clinicopathological documentation of a previously excised pleomorphic adenoma.

The malignant component may look like any type of salivary gland carcinoma and must therefore be classified and graded according to the standard criteria for malignant salivary gland neoplasms [32]. In addition to the tumor type and grade, the extension of malignant growth is important. If confined by the capsule, CPA is designated as intracapsular, in situ, or noninvasive CPA. It has a favorable prognosis, mostly comparable to that of a pleomorphic adenoma.

2.8.4 Comments

1. The grading system for ACC is simple, based on the predominant growth pattern. Patients with tubular (grade I) and cribriform (grade II) patterns have a more favorable prognosis than those with more than 30 % solid growth pattern (grade III). ACC is generally characterized by a slow but relentless progression, but those with solid pattern usually have a more aggressive course, with earlier metastases and poorer survival.

2. In the differential diagnosis of ACC, one must consider polymorphous low-grade adenocarcinoma, epithelial-myoepithelial carcinoma, basal cell carcinoma, and basaloid SCC.

3. Minimally invasive carcinoma ex pleomorphic adenoma, defined as <1.5-mm penetration of malignant cells from the tumor capsule into adjacent tissue, has still a favorable prognosis. If the invasion is greater than 1.5 mm from the tumor capsule, the prognosis is poor, with survival rates at 5, 10, 15, and 20 years ranging from 25 to 65 %, 18 to 50 %, 10 to 35 %, and 0 to 38 %, respectively [28]. Patients with a malignant myoepithelial component may have a less favorable course [32].

Books and Monographs

Barnes L, Eveson JW, Reichart P, Sidransky D (eds) (2005) World Health Organization classification of tumours. Pathology and genetics of head and neck tumours. IARC Press, Lyon

Barnes L (2009) Surgical pathology of the head and neck. Informa Healthcare, New York

Cardesa A, Slootweg P (eds) (2006) Head and neck pathology. Springer, Berlin

Hyams VJ, Batsakis JG, Michaels L (1988) Tumors of the upper respiratory tract and ear, Armed Forces Institute of Pathology Fascicles, 2nd series. American Registry of Pathology Press, Washington DC

Thompson LDR, Wenig BM (2011) Diagnostic pathology. Head and neck. Amirsys, Altona/Manitoba

Articles

1. Gale N, Michaels L, Luzar B et al (2009) Current review on squamous intraepithelial lesions of the larynx. Histopathology 54:639–656
2. Gale N, Kambi V, Michaels L et al (2000) The Ljubljana classification: a practical strategy for the diagnosis of laryngeal precancerous lesions. Adv Anat Pathol 7:240–251

3. van der Waal I (2009) Potentially malignant disorders of the oral and oropharyngeal mucosa; terminology, classification and present concepts of management. Oral Oncol 45:317–323

4. Tilakaratne WM, Sherriff M, Morgan PR, Odell EW (2011) Grading oral epithelial dysplasia: analysis of individual features. J Oral Pathol Med 40:533–540

5. Eversole LR (2009) Dysplasia of the upper aerodigestive tract squamous epithelium. Head Neck Pathol 3:63–68

6. Campisi G, Panzarella V, Giuliani M et al (2007) Human papillomavirus: its identity and controversial role in oral oncogenesis, premalignant and malignant lesions (review). Int J Oncol 30:813–823

7. Gale N, Cardesa A, Zidar N (2006) Larynx and hypopharynx. In: Cardesa A, Slootweg P (eds) Head and neck pathology. Springer, Berlin, pp 198–234

8. Reichart PA, Philipsen HP (2005) Oral erythroplakia -a review. Oral Oncol 41:551–561

9. Begum S, Westra WH (2008) Basaloid squamous cell carcinoma of the head and neck is a mixed variant that can be further resolved by HPV status. Am J Surg Pathol 32:1044–1050

10. Westra WH (2009) The changing face of head and neck cancer in the 21st century: the impact of HPV on the epidemiology and pathology of oral cancer. Head Neck Pathol 3:78–81

11. Marur S, D'Souza G, Westra WH, Forastiere AA (2010) HPV-associated head and neck cancer: a virus-related cancer epidemic. Lancet Oncol 11:781–789

12. Alos L, Moyano S, Nadal A et al (2009) Human papillomaviruses are identified in a subgroup of sinonasal squamous cell carcinomas with favorable outcome. Cancer 115:2701–2709

13. Wiernik G, Millard PR, Haybittle JL (1991) The predictive value of histological classification into degrees of differentiation of squamous cell carcinoma of the larynx and hypopharynx compared with the survival of patients. Histopathology 19:411–417

14. Janot F, Klijanienko J, Russo A et al (1996) Prognostic value of clinicopathologic parameters in head and neck squamous carcinoma: a prospective analysis. Br J Cancer 73:531–538

15. Chiesa F, Mauri S, Tradati N et al (1999) Surfing prognostic factors in head and neck cancer at the millennium. Oral Oncol 35:257–265

16. Thompson LR (2007) Update on nasopharyngeal carcinoma. Head Neck Pathol 1:81–86

17. Franchi A, Moroni M, Massi D et al (2002) Sinonasal undifferentiated carcinoma, nasopharyngeal-type undifferentiated carcinoma, and keratinizing and nonkeratinizing squamous cell carcinoma express different cytokeratin patterns. Am J Surg Pathol 26:1597–1604

18. Jeng YM, Sung MT, Fang CL et al (2002) Sinonasal undifferentiated carcinoma and nasopharyngeal-type undifferentiated carcinoma: two clinically, biologically, and histopathologically distinct entities. Am J Surg Pathol 26:371–376

19. Ejaz A, Wenig BM (2005) Sinonasal undifferentiated carcinoma: clinical and pathologic features and a discussion on classification, cellular differentiation, and differential diagnosis. Adv Anat Pathol 12:134–143

20. Wenig BM (2009) Undifferentiated malignant neoplasms of the sinonasal tract. Arch Pathol Lab Med 133:699–712

21. Barnes L (1986) Intestinal-type adenocarcinoma of the nasal cavity and paranasal sinuses. Am J Surg Pathol 10:192–202

22. Kleinsasser O, Schroeder HG (1988) Adenocarcinomas of the inner nose after exposure to wood dust. Morphological findings and relationships between histopathology and clinical behavior in 79 cases. Arch Otorhinolaryngol 245:1–15

23. Stelow EB, Mills SE, Jo VY, Carlson DL (2010) Adenocarcinoma of the upper aerodigestive tract. Adv Anat Pathol 17:262–269

24. Thompson LD (2010) Intestinal-type sinonasal adenocarcinoma. Ear Nose Throat J 89:16–18

25. Lewis JS, Ferlito A, Gnepp DR, Rinaldo A et al (2011) Terminology and classification of neuroendocrine neoplasms of the larynx. Laryngoscope 121:1187–1193

26. Kusafuka K, Ferlito A, Lewis JS Jr et al (2012) Large cell neuroendocrine carcinoma of the head and neck. Oral Oncol 48:211–215

27. Thompson LD (2009) Olfactory neuroblastoma. Head Neck Pathol 3:252–259

28. Seethala RR (2011) Histologic grading and prognostic biomarkers in salivary gland carcinomas. Adv Anat Pathol 18:29–45

29. Brandwein MS, Ivanov K, Wallace DI et al (2001) Mucoepidermoid carcinoma: a clinicopathologic study of 80 patients with special reference to histological grading. Am J Surg Pathol 25:835–845

30. Luna MA (2006) Salivary mucoepidermoid carcinoma: revisited. Adv Anat Pathol 13:293–307

31. Rapidis AD, Givalos N, Gakiopoulou H et al (2005) Adenoid cystic carcinoma of the head and neck. Clinicopathological analysis of 23 patients and review of the literature. Oral Oncol 41:328–335

32. Katabi N, Gomey D, Klimstra DS et al (2010) Prognostic factors of recurrence in salivary carcinoma ex pleomorphic adenoma, with emphasis on the carcinoma histologic subtype: a clinicopathologic study of 43 cases. Hum Pathol 41:927–934

Tumors of the Lungs and Pleura

3

Nagarjun Rao, Cesar Moran, and Saul Suster

3.1 Introduction

Carcinoma of the lung is a very common malignant tumor. Histological typing of lung tumors has long been a source of controversy in pathology, in great part due to the marked microscopic heterogeneity of these tumors [1–4]. Although the bronchi and lungs may give rise to a wide variety of histopathologic types of malignant epithelial neoplasms, grading of lung cancer is usually restricted to the two most common types of bronchogenic carcinoma included in the latest WHO classification: squamous cell carcinoma and adenocarcinoma. Neuroendocrine carcinomas of the lung constitute a third major group of lung neoplasms that are amenable to grading, as it has been observed that histologic grading of these tumors appears to correlate with their clinical behavior and prognosis [5]. The fourth major category of bronchogenic carcinoma in the WHO classification, large cell carcinoma, is not subject to grading since it is by definition a high-grade neoplasm.

Other less common primary epithelial neoplasms of the bronchus, such as carcinomas of

salivary gland type, usually represent low-grade neoplasms that are rarely amenable to grading [6]. Malignant mesotheliomas of the pleura that have an invariably poor prognosis are by definition high-grade tumors which are usually not graded.

3.2 Squamous Cell Carcinoma

The grading system for squamous cell carcinoma of the bronchus is essentially the same as that for squamous cell cancer in other organs and is based on the extent of microscopic signs of keratinization or the absence of it. A variety of grading systems has been utilized in the past. The American Joint Commission on Cancer (2010) has proposed a 5-tiered grading system that includes the following categories: GX (grade cannot be assessed), G1 (well differentiated), G2 (moderately differentiated), G3 (poorly differentiated), and G4 (undifferentiated). In clinical practice, however, most pathologists have traditionally utilized a three-tiered grading system that includes well-, moderately, and poorly differentiated tumors.

- *Grade 1: Well-Differentiated Squamous Cell Carcinoma*
  These tumors are characterized by prominent keratinization throughout the lesion as well as the presence of discernible intercellular bridges. Keratinization in well-differentiated squamous carcinoma usually adopts the form of "squamous pearls," which appear as concentric laminated aggregates of amorphous,

N. Rao, M.D. • S. Suster, M.D. (✉)
Department of Pathology, Medical College of Wisconsin, Milwaukee, WI, USA
e-mail: ssuster@mcw.edu

C. Moran, M.D.
Department of Pathology,
University of Texas, M.D. Anderson Cancer Center, Houston, TX, USA

I. Damjanov, F. Fan (eds.), *Cancer Grading Manual*,
DOI 10.1007/978-3-642-34516-6_3, © Springer-Verlag Berlin Heidelberg 2013

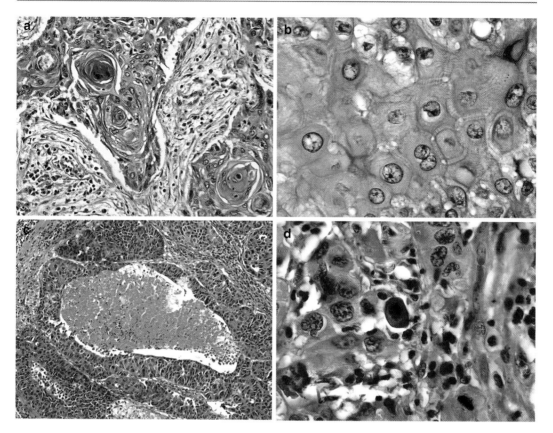

Fig. 3.1 Squamous cell carcinoma of the lung. (**a**) This well-differentiated tumor shows concentric laminated deposits of amorphous, keratinous material ("squamous pearls"). (**b**) Higher magnification of a well-differentiated tumor shows well-formed intercellular bridges. (**c**) Squamous cell carcinoma. This moderately differentiated carcinoma shows central, comedo-like area of necrosis and decrease in size of the tumor cells surrounding the areas of necrosis. (**d**) This poorly differentiated carcinoma shows single-cell keratinization (*center*) surrounded by poorly differentiated neoplastic cells

eosinophilic extracellular keratinous material (Fig. 3.1a). These structures usually are located in the center of large tumor nests that show a "maturation" phenomenon, whereby the central portions of the nests or tumor islands show the most pronounced features of keratinization, while the peripheral portions show a decrease in tumor cell size with the outermost layer being composed of smaller cells with a more basaloid appearance. The cells within the tumor islands show a striking pavement-like architecture, and intercellular bridges resulting from prominence of desmosomal cell junctions due to artifactual cell shrinkage can be readily visualized at the light microscopic level (Fig. 3.1b). The tumor cells are usually characterized by a polygonal shape with very well-defined cell membranes. Clearing of the cytoplasm due to accumulation of glycogen may be present in some tumors. Focal accumulation of mucinous basophilic material that is stained positive with mucicarmine or PAS can be occasionally seen in isolated tumor cells. This feature per se, however, does not change the diagnosis to adenocarcinoma or mucoepidermoid carcinoma if a lung tumor is otherwise showing the typical features of well-differentiated squamous cell carcinoma.

- *Grade 2: Moderately Differentiated Squamous Cell Carcinoma*

These tumors are characterized by a significantly decreased extent of squamous differentiation. Thus, squamous pearls are few or absent, intercellular bridges are more difficult to find and seen only focally, and there is an increased number of smaller, basaloid cells in the tumor cell islands. Central areas of comedo-like necrosis are a common feature in these tumors (Fig. 3.1c). However, the pavement-like appearance of the tumor cells with sharply defined cell borders is generally still preserved.

- *Grade 3: Poorly Differentiated Squamous Cell Carcinoma*
  These tumors are characterized by a lack of squamous differentiation. Intercellular bridges are only rarely seen or not evident at all, and keratin pearls are not present. The tumor cells tend to form confluent sheets or irregular islands or infiltrate the normal tissues as single cells that have bizarre nuclear forms and show marked nuclear pleomorphism. Single-cell keratinization is the most important feature for diagnosis. Individually keratinized cells are usually round and have abundant, slightly refractile eosinophilic cytoplasm (Fig. 3.1d). Their nuclei may be pyknotic or karyolytic resembling apoptotic tumor cells. However, unlike apoptotic cells, they are surrounded by an ample rim of deeply eosinophilic cytoplasm. Small foci of tumor cells showing more advanced features of squamous differentiation can be often identified focally, including polygonal cells with a prominent pavement-like architecture, sharply delimited cell membranes, and small foci of keratinization.

3.2.1   Comments

1. Grading of squamous cell carcinoma is based on the predominant features in a given tumor. For this reason, grading is best reserved for complete resection specimens, since small biopsies may not be representative.
2. A few unusual histologic variants of squamous cell carcinoma of the lung have been described that may not be amenable to grading. These tumors are essentially regarded as high-grade (poorly differentiated) variants of squamous cell carcinoma and include the following microscopic forms:

- Spindle-cell ("sarcomatoid") squamous cell carcinoma
- Basaloid squamous cell carcinoma
- Small cell squamous cell carcinoma
- Lymphoepithelioma-like carcinoma

3. Immunohistochemical markers are of limited value for the diagnosis and grading of squamous cell carcinoma of the lung. Although a variety of immunohistochemical markers have been developed in recent years that have been associated with squamous differentiation (such as high molecular weight cytokeratin CK5/6 or p63), in our experience, their patterns of expression have not been reliable enough to serve a useful purpose for grading of the lesions. However, with the development of targeted therapies mainly aimed at subgroups of adenocarcinoma carrying specific mutations, the International Association for the Study of Lung Cancer (IASLC) recommends the use of these markers, especially in small biopsies and cytology specimens of non-small-cell carcinomas when morphologic features are not diagnostic. In these biopsies, the immunohistochemical stains could help distinguishing squamous cell carcinoma from adenocarcinoma [7].

3.3   Adenocarcinoma of the Lung

The grading system for adenocarcinoma of the lung is primarily based on the ratio of glands to solid elements found within the tumor and in the degree to which these glands resemble normal structures within the lungs (i.e., either bronchioloalveolar spaces or bronchial glands).

- *Grade 1: Well-Differentiated Adenocarcinoma*
  These tumors are characterized by well-formed glandular or acinar structures that comprise more than 90 % of the tumor. The glands are generally well-formed and lined by round or columnar cells with abundant cytoplasm and enlarged nuclei with coarse chromatin pattern and visible nucleoli (Fig. 3.2a). A distinctive form of well-differentiated adenocarcinoma is the "lepidic" pattern adenocarcinoma, previously known as bronchioloalveolar carcinoma. It is character-

ized by the growth of bland-appearing tumor cells along the alveolar walls (Fig. 3.2b). The cells lining the alveolar spaces may be small, round to polygonal with large "hobnail" hyperchromatic nuclei, or may be tall columnar with abundant clear or lightly eosinophilic mucinous cytoplasm (Fig. 3.2c). Please see below for further discussion on lepidic pattern adenocarcinoma and bronchioloalveolar carcinoma.

- *Grade 2: Moderately Differentiated Adenocarcinoma*

  These tumors are characterized by a proliferation of glandular or acinar structures that comprise at least 50 % of the total tumor volume or which no longer closely resemble well-developed glands; i.e., the glands are poorly formed, with poorly developed or only abortive lumens, and are lined by cells showing solid areas with nuclear stratification (Fig. 3.2d). Alternatively, the glands may show well-developed lumens but are lined by highly atypical cells showing marked nuclear pleomorphism, frequent mitoses, and signs of overt anaplasia.

- *Grade 3: Poorly Differentiated Adenocarcinoma*

  These tumors are characterized by a tumor cell proliferation containing fewer glandular

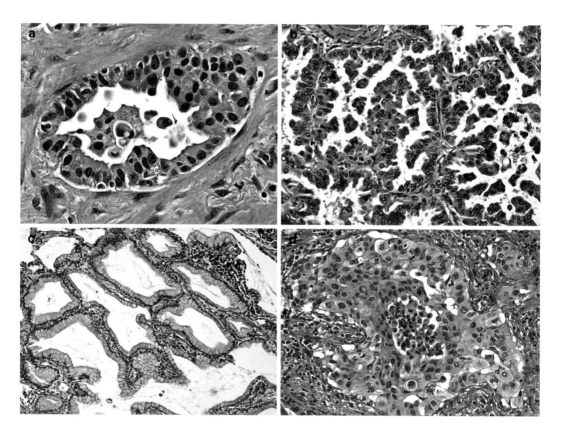

Fig. 3.2 Adenocarcinoma of the lung. (**a**) This well-differentiated tumor consists of well-formed gland lined by a single layer of atypical columnar cells. (**b**) Well-differentiated adenocarcinoma showing characteristic "lepidic" growth pattern (bronchioloalveolar features), with a row of mildly atypical cells continuously lining the alveolar walls. (**c**) Well-differentiated lepidic pattern adenocarcinoma composed of tall, columnar cells with abundant clear mucinous cytoplasm. (**d**) Moderately differentiated adenocarcinoma composed of ill-defined glands with abortive lumina, lined by atypical cells. Tumor also contains solid areas with nuclear stratification. (**e**) Poorly differentiated adenocarcinoma consisting of ill-defined glands lined by highly atypical cells. (**f**) Papillary adenocarcinoma shows complex papillary structures lined by markedly atypical cells. Notice the foci of tumor necrosis in the lumen of the glandular structures. (**g**) Micropapillary adenocarcinoma shows small cell nests within airspaces *without* fibrovascular cores. (**h**) Cribriform adenocarcinoma with cell groups with distinctive roman bridges and necrosis

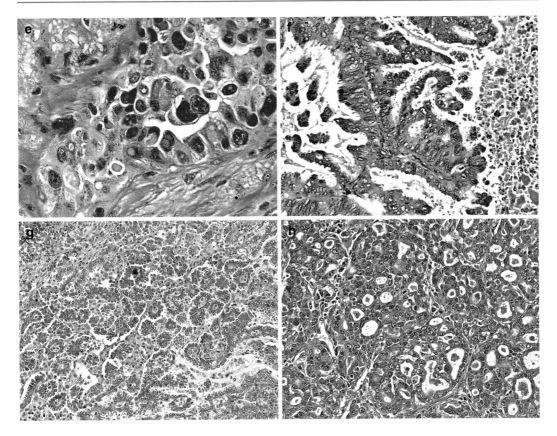

Fig. 3.2 (continued)

or acinar structures (5–50 % of the total tumor volume) and a predominance of solid areas containing frequent mucinous cells (five or more mucin-positive cells in at least 2 high-power fields). The few glands present are usually poorly formed and are lined by highly atypical cells showing marked nuclear pleomorphism (Fig. 3.2e).

3.3.1 Comments

1. Bronchioloalveolar carcinoma (BAC) as a diagnostic category is being reevaluated, partly because of the difficulties associated with applying the histologic features consistently. In the 2004 WHO classification, the term BAC has been reserved for those tumors that grow in a lepidic fashion along preexisting alveolar septa without stromal, pleural, or vascular invasion [4]. This is of clinical significance as tumors of this type which are less than 2.0 cm in size can be cured by simple surgical excision. Those tumors that may have a lepidic spread pattern but show a degree of invasion (stromal, pleural, or vascular) have been characterized as *adenocarcinoma with BAC features*. The International Society for Study of Lung Cancer, along with the American Thoracic Society and the European Respiratory Society (IASLC/ATS/ERS), has recently proposed a new classification scheme and diagnostic criteria for adenocarcinomas, which has essentially deleted the term BAC [7]. The newly proposed terminology recognizing the BAC as a part of the pulmonary adenocarcinoma spectrum has three categories:

   (a) *Adenocarcinoma in situ* is the term used for lesions less than 3 cm in size, formerly characterized as BAC, without stromal, pleural or vascular invasion.

(b) *Minimally invasive adenocarcinomas* are tumors measuring less than 3 cm in size, showing predominantly lepidic growth with stromal invasion measuring less than 5 mm.

(c) *Invasive adenocarcinoma* refers to lesions greater than 3 cm in size or lesions of any size which have a greater than 5-mm stromal invasive component.

It is important to recognize that these criteria can only be applied on resection specimens and lepidic predominant invasive adenocarcinoma cannot be differentiated reliably from adenocarcinoma in situ in small biopsies or cytology specimens. Accordingly, the IASLC recommends that in small biopsies when pure lepidic growth pattern is seen, it should be clarified that an invasive component may not be recognized in a small specimen.

2. The growth of invasive pulmonary adenocarcinoma may occur in several patterns recognized by the WHO classification of 2004 and IASLC/ATS/ERS [3, 7]. These patterns include *lepidic predominant*, *acinar predominant*, *papillary predominant*, *micropapillary predominant*, and *solid predominant with mucin*. It is worthy of notice that *papillary* growth pattern is frequently observed in lepidic predominant adenocarcinoma, in which the papillary structures are seen to invaginate and grow toward the lumen of alveolar spaces. Under these circumstances, the cell population lining the papillae is similar to that of lepidic predominant adenocarcinoma (i.e., cells devoid of significant cytologic atypia or anaplasia). A second, rarer type of tumor has also been described characterized by a predominant papillary growth pattern that has been termed *papillary adenocarcinoma* of the lung [8]. In such tumors, the papillary structures show complex branching and are lined by cells displaying marked nuclear pleomorphism, hyperchromasia, and high mitotic activity (Fig. 3.2f). Such tumors behave in a much more aggressive fashion than bronchioloalveolar carcinoma and are more akin in their behavior to conventional adenocarcinoma of the lung.

3. Several variants of adenocarcinoma of the lung have been described, including the following microscopic forms [3]:
   • Invasive mucinous
   • Colloid
   • Enteric
   • Fetal (low and high grade)

   The majority of these tumors correspond to low-grade, well-differentiated adenocarcinomas, but exceptions also occur. For the fetal adenocarcinoma subgroup, one must specify whether the tumor belongs to the low-grade or the high-grade form.

4. Two growth patterns not mentioned in the 2004 WHO classification may be of clinical significance. These two patterns are the micropapillary and cribriform tumors:
   (a) *Micropapillary pattern* is characterized by the formation of small tufted papillae composed of cells mainly lying freely within air spaces [9]. These papillae are more like little cell nests *without* distinctive fibrovascular cores. Most spaces containing the micropapillae lack a distinctive lining (Fig. 3.2g). These tumors are aggressive, with a propensity for lymphovascular invasion. Individual tumor cells show moderate amounts of eosinophilic cytoplasm with irregular, hyperchromatic nuclei. It is important to remember that the micropapillary pattern may predominate or be the solitary appearance of a tumor, but is more likely to be combined with other patterns.

   (b) *Cribriform pattern* is probably far commoner than recognized [10]. Distinctive features of this tumor subtype include cribriform glandular structures with "roman bridges," dirty comedo-like necrosis, sub- and supranuclear vacuolation, and cystic/mucinous cell components (Fig. 3.2h). It is not yet clear if these tumors have a definite molecular fingerprint. It is important to remember that cribriform adenocarcinoma may overlap morphologically with pulmonary metastases from other locations such as the prostate gland, large bowel, pancreas, breast, and uterus (endometrioid carcinoma), among others.

3.4   Neuroendocrine Carcinomas of the Lung

Neuroendocrine carcinomas of the lungs occur in several clinicopathologic forms, but their classification and grading have been the subject of much debate in recent years [5, 11]. This has been mostly due to the slow trend to abandon older terms such as "carcinoid tumor" and "atypical carcinoid" in favor of the more accurate designation of "neuroendocrine carcinoma" for this family of tumors. The new WHO classification recognizes the existence of a spectrum of lung lesions showing features of neuroendocrine differentiation that can range from very well-differentiated to very poorly differentiated tumors. In deference to established custom, however, the terms carcinoid, atypical carcinoid, and small cell and large cell NEC have been retained in their proposed classification [3].

Another recent proposal has introduced a 4-tiered grading scheme for these tumors that employs terms that are similar to those adopted by the previous WHO schema, with the last category in their classification corresponding to "undifferentiated NEC." We believe the term "undifferentiated" as applied to these tumors should be abandoned since it is contradictory in this setting. The term undifferentiated, by definition, refers to a tumor displaying *no* features of differentiation; whereas the term neuroendocrine carcinoma by definition implies specific evidence of both epithelial and neuroendocrine differentiations. Poorly differentiated NEC would therefore be a more accurate and correct terminology for such tumors. We prefer the use of a more simplified 3-tiered grading system that grades these tumors based on their degrees of differentiation and designates them as low-grade or well-differentiated NEC, intermediate-grade or moderately differentiated NEC, and high-grade or poorly differentiated NEC, respectively.

- *Well-Differentiated Neuroendocrine Carcinoma.* These tumors essentially correspond to what has been previously termed "typical carcinoid" in the literature. The defining criteria are twofold: architectural and cytologic. Architectural criteria include the presence of a well-developed neuroendocrine (or "organoid") pattern of growth in the majority (>80 %) of the tumor, characterized by the arrangement of the tumor cells into well-defined nests, packets, cords, trabeculae, or ribbons usually separated by fibrovascular septa (Fig. 3.3a). Other growth patterns that can be also less frequently observed include the formation of epithelial rosettes, microacinar structures, or tumor cell islands with prominent peripheral palisading of nuclei. Cytologic criteria for well-differentiated NEC include a fairly monotonous tumor cell population composed of relatively small cells with round to oval nuclei showing a characteristically evenly dispersed chromatin pattern ("salt and pepper"), surrounded by a rim of eosinophilic cytoplasm (Fig. 3.3b). Nucleoli are generally absent or inconspicuous, and mitotic activity is usually minimal (<2 mitoses per 10 high-power fields).

- *Moderately Differentiated Neuroendocrine Carcinoma.* These tumors are characterized by at least partial loss of the neuroendocrine growth pattern and more pronounced cytologic atypia with increased mitotic activity. Moderately differentiated NEC essentially corresponds to the tumors previously designated as "*atypical carcinoid*" in the literature. Cellular sheets and islands of relatively monotonous tumor cells that retain, at least focally, a recognizable "organoid" pattern of growth characterize these tumors. Another distinctive feature of these tumors is the presence of central, comedo-like areas of necrosis in many of the tumor cell islands (Fig. 3.3c). Cytologically, the tumors are characterized by cells displaying enlarged nuclei, which can be round or oval, with increase in chromatin pattern, occasional prominent nucleoli, and increased mitotic activity (2–10 mitoses per 10 high-power fields).

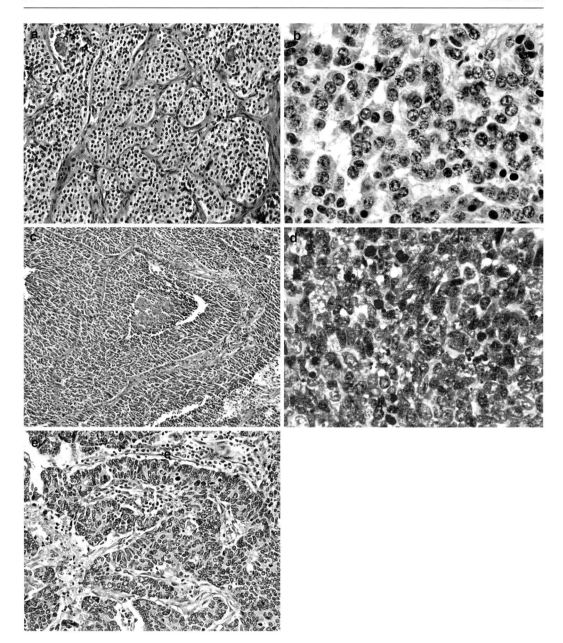

Fig. 3.3 Neuroendocrine carcinoma. (**a**) Well-differentiated neuroendocrine carcinoma ("carcinoid" tumor). The tumor is composed of a monotonous population of small, round tumor cells adopting a prominent "nesting" pattern separated by fibrovascular septa. (**b**) Well-differentiated neuroendocrine carcinoma at higher magnification. One can appreciate the monotonous population of tumor cells with "salt and pepper" nuclear chromatin pattern, absence of prominent nucleoli and mitoses, and indistinct rim of amphophilic to lightly acidophilic cytoplasm. (**c**) Moderately differentiated neuroendocrine carcinoma of the lung ("atypical carcinoid") consists of cells arranged into large lobules with central, comedo-like areas of necrosis. (**d**) Poorly differentiated neuroendocrine carcinoma of the lung, small cell type is composed of cells showing large, hyperchromatic nuclei with "smudged" chromatin. Mitoses are conspicuous. (**e**) Poorly differentiated neuroendocrine carcinoma of the lung, large cell type consists of tumor cells arranged into nests and cords. These cells are large and have abundant cytoplasm adopting a vague "organoid" pattern. The tumor cells demonstrated positivity for chromogranin and synaptophysin by immunohistochemical staining

- *Poorly Differentiated Neuroendocrine Carcinoma*. We currently include two distinct variants within this category: small cell neuroendocrine carcinoma (SCNEC) and large cell neuroendocrine carcinoma (LCNEC). The latter continues to be in dispute, and many authors contend that this tumor likely belongs in a different category, namely, that of large cell/anaplastic carcinoma. It has not yet been determined whether the biologic behavior and response to chemotherapy is the same for the small cell and the large cell variant of NEC [5].

- *Small Cell Neuroendocrine Carcinoma*. SCNEC is generally characterized by sheets of tumor cells with extensive tumor necrosis and without a readily identifiable neuroendocrine architectural growth pattern. The tumor cells are relatively small (compared to large cell or anaplastic carcinoma) and usually have a diameter that is roughly equivalent to or less than that of three small lymphocytes. The cells are characterized by displaying large nuclei with hardly any discernible cytoplasm. The nuclear chromatin is finely dispersed and often appears "smudged," with absent or small nucleoli as visualized in hematoxylin-eosin-stained preparations on routine light microscopy (Fig. 3.3d). Mitotic activity is usually very high, with an average of 10 or more mitoses per 10 high-power fields.

- *Large Cell Neuroendocrine Carcinoma*. LCNEC is currently defined as a lung tumor displaying a readily identifiable neuroendocrine architectural growth pattern (i.e., nest and cords of tumor cells, rosettes, trabeculae) but in which the tumor cells are much larger than in SCNEC (at least double in size), with increased nuclear to cytoplasmic ratio, vesicular chromatin, and prominent nucleoli (Fig. 3.3e). Mitoses are generally frequent and usually exceed 10 per 10 high-power fields. Tumor necrosis is generally prominent and may involve large zones. The diagnosis of LCNEC requires confirmation by immunohistochemistry, i.e., the tumor should be positive for neuroendocrine markers such as chromogranin-A or synaptophysin. Alternatively, one should demonstrate dense-core neurosecretory granules by electron microscopy.

3.4.1 Comments

1. Well-differentiated NEC and moderately differentiated NEC belong to a spectrum of closely related tumors which cannot be always separated one from another on the basis of strict objective criteria. The most important criterion for separating these two tumors is mitotic activity.

2. Although it was initially thought that atypical carcinoid required more than 5 mitoses per 10 high-power fields, that threshold has been recently lowered, and tumors displaying 2 or more mitoses per 10 high-power fields are classified as moderately differentiated NEC.

3. Another important criterion is the presence of necrosis; even focal pinpoint areas of necrosis should strongly raise the consideration of a moderately differentiated NEC when present in an otherwise well-differentiated tumor.

4. Cytologic atypia appears to be less reliable as a single criterion for separating these tumors. It is recommended that mitoses be counted in the areas of higher mitotic activity using a 40× objective with an eyepiece that has a field-of-view number of 20 (the area viewed in 1 high-power field should equal 0.2 mm^2 or 2 mm^2 for 10 high-power fields).

5. Poorly differentiated neuroendocrine carcinomas may also show a variable admixture of small and large cell types within the same tumor. Such cases are designated as mixed small/large cell neuroendocrine carcinoma.

6. It must be noted that a subset of non-small-cell carcinomas of the lung may display immunohistochemical or ultrastructural features of neuroendocrine differentiation despite not showing a "neuroendocrine" architectural growth pattern. Neuroendocrine differentiation has been demonstrated by immunohistochemistry in up to 20 % of squamous cell carcinomas, adenocarcinomas, and large cell carcinomas. These tumors have been collectively referred to as "non-small-cell lung cancer with neuroendocrine differentiation." Their exact relationship to the group of LCNEC is still poorly defined and remains a controversial topic.

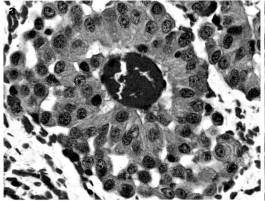
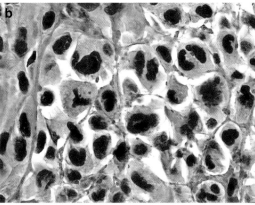

Fig. 3.4 Malignant mesothelioma. (**a**) Epithelioid meso-thelioma is composed of large, round to polygonal tumor cells with abundant cytoplasm and minimal nuclear atypia. (**b**) Tumor cells have high-grade nuclei showing marked nuclear pleomorphism, hyperchromatism, and abnormal mitoses

7. In approximately 5–7 % of all tumor cases, even the experts in lung cancer pathology cannot agree on whether a tumor is a SCNEC or a non-small-cell lung carcinoma [11]. These tumors usually belong to the high-grade category.

3.5   Malignant Mesothelioma

Malignant mesothelioma is defined as a neoplastic proliferation of mesothelial cells originating from the visceral or parietal pleura [12]. Three basic types are described:
• Epithelioid mesothelioma
• Sarcomatoid ("spindle cell") mesothelioma
• Biphasic ("mixed epithelioid/sarcomatoid") mesothelioma

Less common variants of malignant mesothelioma include the desmoplastic, deciduoid, lymphohistiocytoid, clear cell, small cell, and pleomorphic variants [13, 14]. These mesotheliomas must be distinguished from metastatic malignant tumors involving the pleura and other less common primary pleural tumors [15]. Malignant mesothelioma may also resemble reactive mesothelial proliferative lesions [16].

Because of the uniformly dismal prognosis of malignant mesotheliomas, these tumors commonly are not graded. The vast majority of malignant mesotheliomas (i.e., epithelioid malignant meso-thelioma) actually display low-grade cytologic features and are characterized by a relatively bland-appearing, well-differentiated population of cells that closely resemble their benign counterpart (Fig. 3.4a). The architectural growth pattern of these tumors, namely, the formation of tubulopapillary structures, is also closely reminiscent of benign reactive mesothelium. The cells in sarcomatoid mesothelioma, on the other hand, no longer resemble normal mesothelium and rather can mimic a spindle-cell sarcoma due to their elongated shape and atypia. The latter could be conceptually regarded as a poorly differentiated or cytologically high-grade variant of malignant mesothelioma. The differences in behavior and prognosis for these tumors, however, are minimal due to their uniformly dismal outcome making this distinction of little clinical significance. In rare instances, epithelioid malignant meso-thelioma may form solid sheets composed of highly atypical and even anaplastic tumor cells with increased nuclear to cytoplasmic ratios, marked nuclear pleomorphism, and frequent mitotic figures; such tumors de facto represent a cytologically high-grade, poorly differentiated variant of epithelioid malignant mesothelioma (Fig. 3.4b).

Books and Monographs

American Joint Commission on Cancer (2010) Cancer staging manual, 7th edn. Springer, Berlin

Leslie KO, Wick MR (2011) Practical pulmonary pathology. A diagnostic approach. Saunders Elsevier, Philadelphia

Moran CA, Suster S (2010) Tumors and tumor-like conditions of the lung and pleura. Saunders Elsevier, Philadelphia

Travis WD, Brambilla E, M ller-Hermelink HK, Harris CC (eds) (2004) World Health Organization classification of tumours. Pathology and genetics of tumours of the lung, pleura, thymus and heart. IARC Press, Lyon

Articles

1. Yesner R (1981) The dynamic histopathologic spectrum of lung cancer. Yale J Biol Med 54:447–456
2. Dunnill MS, Gatter KC (1986) Cellular heterogeneity in lung cancer. Histopathology 10:461–475
3. Travis WD (2011) Pathology of lung cancer. Clin Chest Med 32:669–692
4. Beasley MB, Brambilla E, Travis WD (2005) The 2004 World Health Organization classification of lung tumors. Semin Roentgenol 40:90–97
5. Huang Q, Muzitansky A, Mark EJ (2002) Pulmonary neuroendocrine carcinomas: a review of 234 cases and a statistical analysis of 50 cases treated at one institution using a simple clinicopathologic classification. Arch Pathol Lab Med 126:545–553
6. Moran CA (1995) Primary salivary gland-type tumors of the lung. Semin Diagn Pathol 12:123–139
7. Travis WD, Brambilla E, Noguchi M et al (2011) International Association for the Study of Lung Cancer/American Thoracic Society/European Respiratory Society international multidisciplinary classification of lung adenocarcinoma. J Thorac Oncol 6:244–285
8. Aida S, Shimazaki H, Sato K et al (2004) Prognostic analysis of pulmonary adenocarcinoma subclassification with special consideration of papillary and bronchioloalveolar types. Histopathology 45:468–476
9. Amin MB, Tamboli B, Merchant SH et al (2002) Micropapillary component in lung adenocarcinoma – a distinctive histologic feature with possible prognostic significance. Am J Surg Pathol 26:358–364
10. Luevano A, Rao N, Mackinnon AC, Suster S (2012) Cribriform adenocarcinoma of the lung: clinicopathologic, immunohistochemical and molecular study of 15 cases. Mod Pathol 25:483A
11. Travis WD (2012) Update on small cell carcinoma and its differentiation from squamous cell carcinoma and other non-small cell carcinomas. Mod Pathol 25:S18–S30
12. Robinson BW, Musk AW, Lake RA (2005) Malignant mesothelioma. Lancet 366:397–408
13. Ordóñez NG (2012) Mesotheliomas with small cell features: report of eight cases. Mod Pathol 25:689–698
14. Ordóñez NG (2012) Pleomorphic mesothelioma: report of 10 cases. Mod Pathol 25:1011–1022
15. Granville L, Laga AC, Allen TC et al (2005) Review and update of uncommon primary pleural tumors: a practical approach to diagnosis. Arch Pathol Lab Med 129:1428–1443
16. Cagle PT, Churg A (2005) Differential diagnosis of benign and malignant mesothelial proliferations on pleural biopsies. Arch Pathol Lab Med 129:1421–1427

Tumors of the Thymus

4

Saul Suster and Cesar Moran

4.1 Introduction

Primary thymic epithelial neoplasms represent the most common type of tumors of the anterior mediastinum. These tumors have been a source of major controversy over the years due to their difficulties for histopathologic typing and often unpredictable biologic behavior. Unlike malignant epithelial neoplasms arising at other organs, these tumors were felt for many years to be unsuitable for histologic grading. In fact, the latest WHO schema for the classification of thymic epithelial neoplasms does not mention grading for these tumors at all. More recent observations, however, have demonstrated that thymic epithelial neoplasms form part of a continuous spectrum of lesions that may closely resemble their parent organ at the one end or be very poorly differentiated at the other extreme [1]. Based on these observations, a novel conceptual approach was recently introduced for the classification of thymic epithelial neoplasms that is based on the histologic degree of differentiation of the lesions [2]. The histologic grading of these tumors is based on the premise that these lesions can range from well-differentiated to moderately differentiated to poorly differentiated neoplasms. This is supported by the observation of tumor progression in thymoma whereby recurrences show transformation of a low-grade histologic type to that of a higher-grade histology [3]. The degree of differentiation in any given tumor will depend on the presence or absence of the organotypical features of differentiation of the thymus and on the degree of cytological atypia displayed by the tumor cells (see Table 4.1).

Tumors displaying most or all of the organotypical features of thymic differentiation and

S. Suster, M.D. (⊠)
Department of Pathology, Medical College of Wisconsin, Milwaukee, WI, USA
e-mail: ssuster@mcw.edu

C. Moran, M.D.
Department of Pathology,
University of Texas, M.D. Anderson Cancer Center, Houston, TX, USA

Table 4.1 Organotypical features of differentiation of the normal mature thymus of childhood and the normal involuted thymus of the adult

Normal mature thymus of childhood or adolescence

Thick capsule with internal lobulation separated by fibrous septae

Dual (epithelial/lymphoid) cell population with variable numbers of immature T-lymphocytes

Dilated perivascular spaces

Areas of "medullary" differentiation

Absence of cytological features of malignancy

Normal involuted thymus of the adult

Thick capsule with internal lobulation

Spindle cell population devoid of cytologic atypia

Scant immature T-lymphocytes

Rosette-like epithelial structures

Cysts and glandular structures

Adapted by permission from Suster S, Moran CA (2003) The mediastinum. In: Weidner N, Cote RJ, Suster S, Weiss LM (eds) Modern surgical pathology. W.B. Saunders Co, Philadelphia, pp 439–499

I. Damjanov, F. Fan (eds.), *Cancer Grading Manual*,
DOI 10.1007/978-3-642-34516-6_4, © Springer-Verlag Berlin Heidelberg 2013

absence of cytological atypia are categorized as low-grade or well-differentiated thymic epithelial neoplasms (also designated, by convention, thymoma), tumors retaining only some of the organotypical features of the thymus but displaying mild to moderate cytologic atypia correspond to moderately differentiated thymic epithelial neoplasms (atypical thymomas), and tumors showing total loss of the organotypical features of the thymus and displaying overt cytologic evidence of malignancy correspond to high-grade or poorly differentiated thymic epithelial neoplasms (also designated, by convention, thymic carcinomas) [2, 4]. It is to be noted that the grading of these tumors is based on a combination of architectural and cytological parameters as observed on routine microscopy on hematoxylin-eosin-stained slides and does not require the use of special stains or other ancillary techniques.

4.2   Well-Differentiated Thymic Epithelial Neoplasms (Thymoma)

The diagnosis of well-differentiated thymoma is based on the identification of the organotypical features of differentiation of the thymus and the absence of significant cytological atypia in the tumor cells. The organotypical features of the thymus can vary depending on whether the tumor cells are attempting to recapitulate the normal, mature thymus of infants and adolescents or whether they resemble the normal involuted thymus of the adult (see Table 4.1). In general, the better-differentiated tumors are characterized by a thick capsule, fibrous bands with prominent lobulation, and an overwhelming population of immature T-lymphocytes admixed with the neoplastic epithelial cells, thus closely resembling the thymic cortex in children and adolescents. Dilated perivascular spaces and so-called areas of "medullary" differentiation are other frequent features seen in these lesions. The neoplastic epithelial cells are characterized by large vesicular nuclei with prominent eosinophilic nucleoli and are surrounded by an indistinct rim of abundant lightly eosinophilic or amphophilic cytoplasm (Fig. 4.1). Mitoses are not a feature of the neoplastic cells, although in some cases they may be relatively frequent in the surrounding immature T-lymphocytic population. Well-differentiated thymomas that resemble the normal involuted thymus of the adult are composed predominantly of a monotonous population of oval to spindle cells admixed with variable numbers of T-lymphocytes. The neoplastic spindle cells are

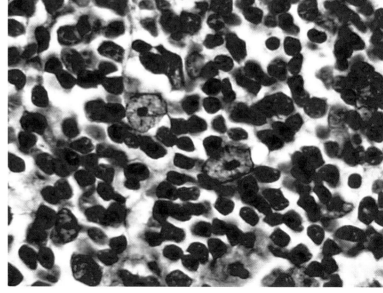

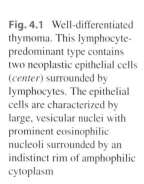

Fig. 4.1 Well-differentiated thymoma. This lymphocyte-predominant type contains two neoplastic epithelial cells (*center*) surrounded by lymphocytes. The epithelial cells are characterized by large, vesicular nuclei with prominent eosinophilic nucleoli surrounded by an indistinct rim of amphophilic cytoplasm

Fig. 4.2 Well-differentiated thymoma of spindle cell type. The tumor is composed of cells with oval to spindle nuclei. The nuclei have dispersed chromatin and absent or inconspicuous nucleoli. There is no mitotic activity

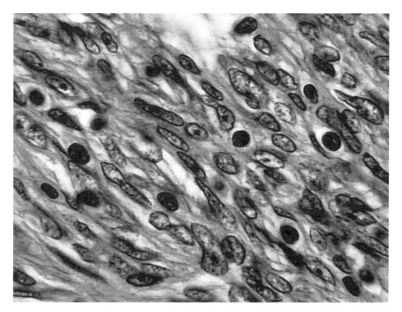

characterized by bland-appearing oval nuclei with dispersed chromatin and inconspicuous nucleoli surrounded by a scant rim of lightly eosinophilic cytoplasm (Fig. 4.2). The cells are devoid of nuclear pleomorphism or mitotic activity.

4.3 Moderately Differentiated Thymic Epithelial Neoplasms (Atypical Thymoma)

These tumors are characterized by partial loss of the organotypical features of differentiation of the normal thymus, with mild to moderate increase in cytologic atypia of the neoplastic epithelial cells. Atypical thymoma may be composed of round/polygonal or oval/spindle cells. The majority of these tumors, however, are composed of large, round to polygonal epithelial cells admixed with scattered T-lymphocytes. Architecturally, the tumors may show some of the organotypical features commonly found in thymoma, such as a thick capsule, lobulation, and perivascular spaces (Fig. 4.3). The tumor cells, however, are much larger than in conventional thymomas, and the cells are characteristically surrounded by abundant eosinophilic cytoplasm showing well-defined cell borders. The nuclei are also larger than in thymomas and

show an increase in chromatin deposition with often prominent eosinophilic nucleoli (Fig. 4.4). Occasional mitotic figures can be observed in the epithelial cells; mitoses may be typical or more rarely atypical but are usually not numerous (usually <2 per 10 high-power fields). A distinctive feature of these tumors is the presence of well-defined cell membranes in the epithelial tumor cells which contrasts with the indistinct cytoplasmic cell borders seen in thymoma. The polygonal shape of the cells and the sharply outlined, thick cell membranes often impart an epidermoid appearance to these tumors. In fact, microscopic foci displaying abrupt squamous differentiation are a frequent finding in these lesions. The tumors are distinguished by a highly cohesive growth pattern forming solid sheets of tumor cells, in contrast to the discohesive growth pattern of well-differentiated thymomas that are characterized by isolated tumor cells separated by abundant lymphocytes. Perivascular spaces are often numerous and show a tendency to display prominent peripheral palisading of tumor cells around the lumen of the vessels. Atypical thymomas composed of oval or spindle cells are also characterized by increase of their nuclear size, with a heavy chromatin pattern, frequent eosinophilic nucleoli, and occasional mitotic figures.

Fig. 4.3 Moderately differentiated thymic epithelial neoplasm (atypical thymoma). Tumor cells form solid sheets around the dilated thin-walled blood vessels. Epithelial cells predominate, but there are also scattered lymphocytes

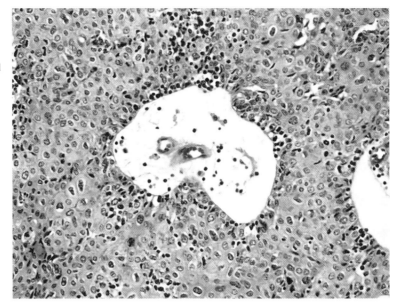

Fig. 4.4 Moderately differentiated thymic epithelial neoplasm (atypical thymoma). Higher magnification of the tumor showing large round to polygonal cells with sharply defined cell membranes and enlarged, hyperchromatic nuclei with occasionally prominent eosinophilic nucleoli

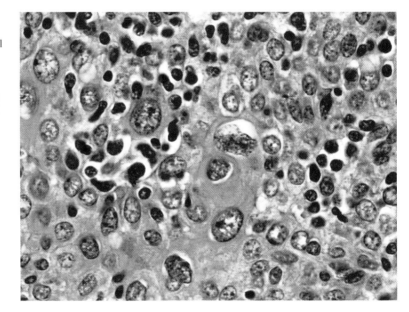

4.4 Poorly Differentiated Thymic Epithelial Neoplasms (Thymic Carcinoma)

These tumors are defined as having lost the characteristic organotypical features of the thymus and by displaying overt cytologic evidence of malignancy. Thymic carcinomas can display a wide variety of microscopic appearances and may closely resemble carcinomas of other organs [4, 5].

As such, they represent essentially a diagnosis of exclusion requiring strict clinical and radiographic demonstration of the absence of a primary tumor elsewhere. A large number of histologic varieties of thymic carcinoma have been described. In the study by Suster and Rosai [4], the tumors could be divided based on their morphologic features into those of low-grade and high-grade histology. It remains debatable whether some of the tumors in the low-grade category may not be best

Fig. 4.5 Poorly differentiated thymic epithelial neoplasm. This tumor has the microscopic features of a mucoepidermoid carcinoma. It is composed of islands of polygonal, epidermoid tumor cells containing cystic luminal spaces filled with mucin. There is no resemblance to the normal thymus

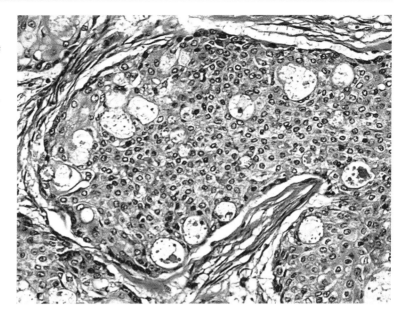

Fig. 4.6 Lymphoepithelioma-like carcinoma. The tumor shows islands of primitive-appearing cells with central comedo-like areas of necrosis

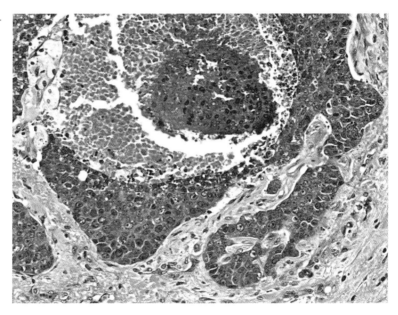

reclassified as moderately differentiated thymic epithelial neoplasms (atypical thymoma), a category that was not yet acknowledged at the time of publication of that study [4]. In any event, the several categories of thymic carcinoma have been described as follows:

- *Squamous cell carcinoma.* These tumors may be well differentiated or poorly differentiated and resemble squamous cell carcinoma in other sites. They, however, usually retain a lobular growth pattern typical of other thymomas.

- *Mucoepidermoid carcinoma* (Fig. 4.5). These tumors resemble the homonymous tumors of the salivary glands and may present likewise as either well-differentiated, moderately differentiated, or poorly differentiated carcinomas.
- *Lymphoepithelioma-like carcinoma* (Fig. 4.6). These tumors resemble the homonymous tumors of the nasopharynx.
- *Clear cell carcinoma* (Fig. 4.7). These tumors are composed of clear cells containing abundant glycogen in their clear cytoplasm.

Fig. 4.7 Clear cell carcinoma of the thymus. The tumor is composed of clear cells but also shows keratinization. The tumor did not display any of the organotypical features of differentiation of the normal thymus

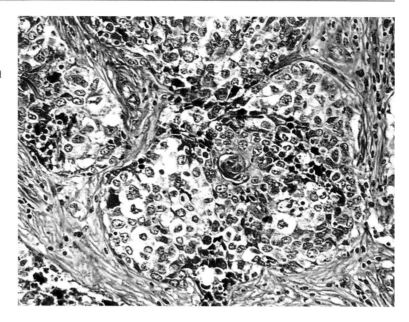

- *Basaloid carcinoma.* These tumors resemble basal cell carcinomas of the skin and are composed of uniform round to oval cells with hyperchromatic nuclei and prominent peripheral palisading.
- *Mucinous adenocarcinoma.* These tumors resemble mucin-secreting tumors in other parts of the body [6].
- *Adenoid cystic carcinoma.* These tumors resemble homonymous tumors of salivary glands [7].
- *Small cell neuroendocrine carcinoma.* These tumors are indistinguishable from homonymous pulmonary carcinomas.
- *Sarcomatoid carcinoma.* This tumor type, is composed predominantly of spindle cells, suggesting the diagnosis of a mesenchymal malignancy. Foci of epithelial differentiation may be scant but are useful for the final diagnosis.
- *Anaplastic carcinoma.* This tumor type, is usually composed of pleomorphic cells, showing almost no signs of differentiation.

The cytologic and architectural features of these tumors are essentially similar to those of their counterparts in other organs [5]. In general, thymic carcinoma is characterized by marked cytologic atypia, increased mitotic activity, and frequent areas of necrosis and vascular invasion.

4.4.1 Comments

1. Great controversy has existed in the literature regarding the best approach to the classification of thymic epithelial neoplasms. The controversy has centered in recent years mainly on the issue of whether morphology alone is sufficient to predict the clinical behavior of these tumors. The consensus of opinion seems to be that morphology alone, particularly for the better-differentiated (low-grade) variants of thymic epithelial neoplasms, is an unreliable predictor of clinical behavior and that staging (i.e., the status of capsular integrity) is the most important parameter for the prediction of biologic behavior in these tumors.
2. The identification of moderately differentiated tumors (atypical thymoma) may be of significance due to their higher incidence of capsular invasion, tendency for earlier recurrence, and potential for transformation into a higher-grade malignancy [1, 4].
3. Several series of thymomas showing uncommon microscopic features have been published during the last few years. For example, there are papers describing thymomas with prominent papillary and pseudopapillary features and so-called adenomatoid spindle cell thymomas, just to mention a few [8, 9]. It is

important to recognize these variants and not to confuse them with thymic carcinomas. Also it is worth remembering, as pointed out in the study of invasive spindle cell thymomas (WHO type A), "that histologic features do not correlate with invasion or encapsulation because all thymomas, regardless of their histologic type are capable of invasion" [10].

Books and Monographs

Rosai J (1999) Histological typing of tumors of the thymus. World Health Organization international histological classification of tumours, 2nd edn. Springer, Berlin

Weidner N, Cote RJ, Suster S, Weiss LM (eds) (2009) Modern surgical pathology, 2nd edn. Saunders Elsevier, Philadelphia

Articles

1. Suster S, Moran CA (1996) Primary thymic epithelial neoplasms with combined features of thymoma and thymic carcinoma. A clinicopathologic study of 22 cases. Am J Surg Pathol 20:1469–1480
2. Suster S, Moran CA (1999) Thymoma, atypical thymoma and thymic carcinoma. A novel conceptual approach to the classification of neoplasms of thymic epithelium. Am J Clin Pathol 111:826–833
3. Suster S, Moran CA (1999) Primary thymic epithelial neoplasms. Spectrum of differentiation and histologic features. Semin Diagn Pathol 16:2–17
4. Suster S, Rosai J (1991) Thymic carcinoma. A clinicopathologic study of 60 cases. Cancer 67: 1025–1032
5. Suster S, Moran CA (1998) Thymic carcinoma: spectrum of differentiation and histologic types. Pathology 30:111–122
6. Ra SH, Fishbei MC, Baruch-Oren T et al (2007) Mucinous adenocarcinomas of the thymus: report of 2 cases and review of the literature. Am J Surg Pathol 31:1330–1338
7. Di Tommaso L, Kuhn E, Kurrer M et al (2007) Thymic tumor with adenoid cystic carcinomalike features: a clinicopathologic study of 4 cases. Am J Surg Pathol 31:1161–1167
8. Kalhor N, Suster S, Moran CA (2011) Spindle cell thymomas (WHO type A) with prominent papillary and pseudopapillary features: a clinicopathologic and immunohistochemical study of 10 cases. Am J Surg Pathol 35:372–377
9. Weissferdt A, Kalhor N, Suster S, Moran CA (2010) Adenomatoid spindle cell thymomas: a clinicopathological and immunohistochemical study of 20 cases. Am J Surg Pathol 34:1544–1549
10. Moran CA, Kalhor N, Suster S (2010) Invasive spindle cell thymomas (WHO type A): a clinicopathologic correlation of 41 cases. Am J Clin Pathol 134: 793–798

Tumors of the Digestive System

5

William L. Neumann and Robert M. Genta

5.1 Introduction

Tissue from the alimentary canal, the hepatobiliary system, and the pancreas accounts for a significant portion of the day-to-day surgical pathology material in most diagnostic pathology laboratories. While many of the tumors encountered in these specimens are microscopically identical to homonymous tumors in other parts of the body and are graded similarly, some are unique to the gastrointestinal system. This chapter reviews the grading of the most common neoplasms of the digestive system. Several grading systems exist. In this chapter, we essentially adhere to the schemas agreed upon at the editorial and consensus conference of the International Agency of Research for Cancer (Lyon) December 2009 and published as the World Health Organization (WHO) *Classification of Tumours of the Digestive System* (Bosman et al. 2010).

Because the same grading criteria can be applied to the same types of tumors throughout the digestive tract, we will first provide general criteria and then discuss their application and differences to each organ. Organ-specific tumors

W.L. Neumann, M.D. • R.M. Genta, M.D. (✉)
University of Texas Southwestern Health Science
Center at Dallas and Miraca Life Sciences,
Dallas, TX, USA
e-mail: robert.genta@utsouthwestern.edu

will be discussed exclusively in the pertinent sections. As a general rule, if there is intratumoral heterogeneity, the highest-grade component should be reported.

5.2 Grading Criteria

5.2.1 Squamous Cell Carcinoma

Squamous cell carcinomas of the digestive tract, like other squamous cancers elsewhere, may be graded based upon the relative proportions of keratinization, intercellular bridges, and primitive basal cells [1]. A 4-grade system, in which the tumors are classified as well differentiated (grade 1), moderately differentiated (grade 2), poorly differentiated (grade 3), or undifferentiated (grade 4), is widely accepted (Bosman et al. 2010):

- *Grade 1, well-differentiated squamous cell carcinoma.* Well-differentiated squamous cell carcinoma is composed of cells that closely resemble those found in normal squamous epithelium. Neoplastic cells in the center of tumor nests appear more mature and have more abundant eosinophilic cytoplasm in comparison to the cells in the periphery. Intercellular bridges are abundant, and keratin pearls, consisting of extracellular keratin arranged in whorls, are frequent. There is a paucity of compact basaloid cells.

I. Damjanov, F. Fan (eds.), *Cancer Grading Manual*,
DOI 10.1007/978-3-642-34516-6_5, © Springer-Verlag Berlin Heidelberg 2013

Fig. 5.1 A focal keratin pearl is seen in this otherwise poorly differentiated squamous cell carcinoma

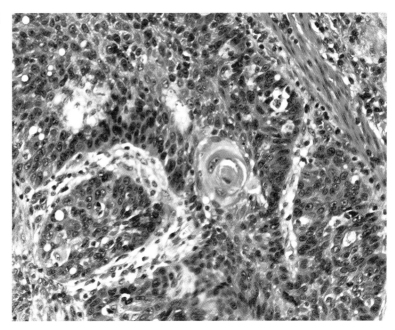

- *Grade 2, moderately differentiated squamous cell carcinoma.* A moderately differentiated tumor has irregular nests and a higher proportion of primitive basal cells than well-differentiated tumors. The tumor cells, although still recognizable as squamous, have less cytoplasm and form less keratin than those in well-differentiated tumors. Intercellular bridges are retained although they are less conspicuous than a well-differentiated tumor.
- *Grade 3, poorly differentiated squamous cell carcinoma.* Poorly differentiated squamous cell carcinoma may consist of sheets, nests, or strands of tumor cells that often exhibit marked nuclear pleomorphism. Individual tumor cells invading the surrounding stroma are not uncommon. Unlike lower-grade squamous cell carcinomas, both keratinization and intercellular bridges are rare and may be confined to only a few cells (Fig. 5.1). These tumors are often mitotically active with numerous atypical mitotic figures.
- *Grade 4, undifferentiated squamous cell carcinoma.* These tumors lack morphologic features

of squamous differentiation but express squamous epithelial markers. Neuroendocrine markers should be negative.

5.2.2 Adenocarcinoma

According to the guidelines of the *WHO Classification of Tumours of the Digestive System* (Bosman et al. 2010), which we are following in this chapter, adenocarcinomas are graded by the proportion of fully formed glands seen histologically and are generally classified as well differentiated, moderately differentiated, or poorly differentiated:

- *Well-differentiated carcinomas.* Over 95 % of the tumor consists of regularly shaped, cystic, or tubular glands with open lumina. The tumor cells are cuboidal or columnar with a variable amount of eosinophilic or clear cytoplasm. The nuclei are vesicular with a coarse chromatin pattern.
- *Moderately differentiated.* Glands compose 50–95 % of the tumor (Fig. 5.2a). The tumor cells in nonglandular areas may be arranged in

Fig. 5.2 Adenocarcinoma. (**a**) A moderately differentiated adenocarcinoma, the majority of which forms glands. (**b**) Poorly differentiated adenocarcinoma composed of signet ring cells

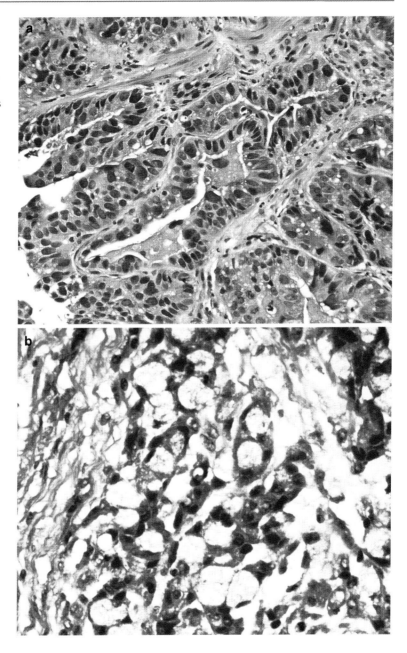

irregular clusters or solid nests. The glandular regions may be cribriform or show extensive nuclear stratification.

- *Poorly differentiated.* Glands comprise less than 50 % of the tumor mass. Most of the neoplastic cells are arranged into solid sheets, nests, or cords. The glands are poorly formed, and tumor cells show considerable pleomorphism. Single cells invading the adjacent tissue can also be found and may exhibit signet ring cell morphology (Fig. 5.2b).

5.2.3 Neuroendocrine Neoplasms

Neoplasms with neuroendocrine differentiation include neuroendocrine tumors (NET) and neuroendocrine carcinomas (NEC). Tumors with an exocrine and an endocrine component, with one component exceeding 30 %, are classified as mixed adenoneuroendocrine carcinomas (MANEC) [2].

Grading is based on morphological criteria (with some variations for each organ) and the assessment of proliferation fraction as established by the European Neuroendocrine Tumor Society (ENTS) scheme [3, 4]. The grading system based on proliferation requires mitotic counts in at least 50 high-power fields (HPF) and Ki-67 labeling index of 500–2,000 cells counted in areas of highest activity [5, 6]:

- *Grade 1*. Mitotic count of <2 per 10 HPF and/or a Ki-67 index ≤2 %
- *Grade 2*. Mitotic count of 2–20 per 10 HPF and/or Ki-67 index of 3–20 %
- *Grade 3 (neuroendocrine carcinoma or NEC)*. Mitotic count >20 per 10 HPF and/or Ki-67 index >20 %

5.2.4 Gastrointestinal Stromal Tumors

Gastrointestinal stromal tumors (GISTs), possibly related to the interstitial cells of Cajal, occur throughout the gastrointestinal tract or rarely at extraintestinal sites [7–10]. The most common site is the stomach followed by the small intestine. These tumors are most often composed of spindle cells, although a minority is epithelioid or rarely of mixed type (Fig. 5.3). Various systems formulated to prognosticate clinical behavior of GISTs have been proposed over the years. Most of these systems have been based upon tumor location, size, and mitotic count. One such system for GISTs originating in the stomach and small intestine was developed by the AFIP [8–10], was independently validated [11], and has been adopted by the WHO (Table 5.1). As understanding of these tumors continues to evolve, future systems will likely incorporate protein kinase KIT, platelet-derived growth factor receptor A (PDGFRA), and succinate dehydrogenase (SDH) mutation status in addition to other markers to predict both clinical behavior and response to therapeutic agents [12–14].

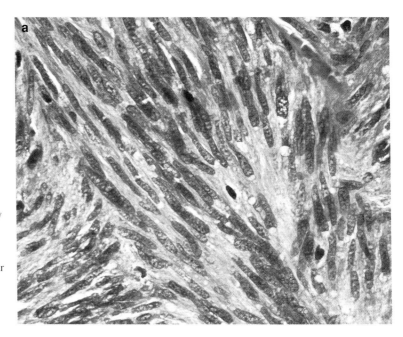

Fig. 5.3 Gastrointestinal stromal tumor (GIST). (**a**) Typical GIST morphology consisting of spindle cells with paranuclear vacuoles, abundant eosinophilic cytoplasm, and foci of nuclear palisading reminiscent of a schwannoma. (**b**) GIST with epithelioid features such as round nuclei

Fig. 5.3 (continued)

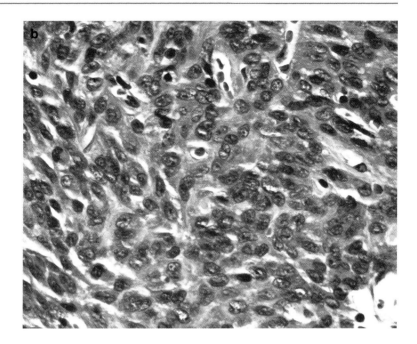

Table 5.1 Armed Forces Institute of Pathology prognostic schema for gastrointestinal stromal tumors

Tumor parameters			Progressive disease during follow-up (% of patients)	
Prognostic group	Size (cm)	Mitotic rate (per 50 HPFs)	Gastric	Small intestinal
1	≤2	≤5	0	0
2	>2≤5	≤5	1.9	4.3
3a	>5≤10	≤5	3.6	24
3b	>10	≤5	12	52
4	≤2	>5	0	50[a]
5	>2≤5	>5	16	73
6a	>5≤10	>5	55	85
6b	>10	>5	86	90

Modified from Miettinen M, Fletcher CDM et al (2010) In: Bosman FT, Carneiro F, Hruban RH, Theise ND (eds) World Health Organization classification of tumours. WHO classification of tumours of the digestive system, 4th edn. IARC Press, Lyon
HPF high-power field
[a]Based on data with few cases

5.2.5   Sarcomas

Primary sarcomas of the gastrointestinal tract are rare but may develop in any organ as mesenchymal tissue is ubiquitous. These tumors are graded similarly to their homonymous counterparts as described in Chap. 13.

5.3   Organ-Specific Tumors

5.3.1   Esophagus

Squamous cell carcinoma and adenocarcinoma represent, by far, the two most common tumors of the esophagus [1]. In North America and Europe, the incidence of adenocarcinomas originating in Barrett esophagus has markedly increased, but in China squamous carcinoma still represents the most common form of esophageal carcinoma [15].

Esophageal squamous cell carcinoma is graded according to the scheme provided above. Most tumors are well or moderately well differentiated. Rare variants include the following:

- *Verrucous carcinoma.* This is a very well-differentiated keratinizing tumor with minimal cytologic atypia.
- *Spindle cell carcinoma.* This tumor, known also as sarcomatoid carcinoma, pseudosarcoma, or carcinosarcoma is histologically biphasic consisting of a high-grade spindle cell component and an epithelial-like component.
- *Basaloid carcinoma.* This aggressive variant resembles homonymous tumors in the upper gastrointestinal tract and is composed of basaloid cells forming solid nests with peripheral palisading along the basement membrane. Some tumors include areas of conventional squamous cell carcinoma, but even so their grade is based on their least differentiated components.

Esophageal adenocarcinoma arises predominantly from metaplastic (Barrett's) mucosa in the distal esophagus. Very rare cases are associated with inlet patches. Adenocarcinoma in Barrett's mucosa develops through a cascade of premalignant lesions (dysplasia) which can be classified in biopsies as follows: negative for dysplasia, indefinite for dysplasia, low-grade dysplasia, high-grade dysplasia, and intramucosal adenocarcinoma. The nuances of this scheme and the controversies surrounding its practical value are beyond the scope of this chapter. Grading of esophageal invasive adenocarcinoma uses the 3-tiered system described earlier.

Gastrointestinal stromal tumors (*GISTs*) of the esophagus are rare and are not covered by the prognostic scheme detailed above. However, most are incidentally detected when they are small and have a benign prognosis.

5.3.2   Stomach

Gastric adenocarcinoma is the most common malignant tumor of the stomach. Several microscopic subtypes are recognized such as tubular, papillary, mucinous, poorly cohesive, mixed, and hepatoid [16]. The 3-tiered scheme outlined previously applies primarily to the tubular and papillary carcinomas. The poorly cohesive type, which includes signet ring cell carcinoma, is by definition poorly differentiated.

Gastric NETs are classified in three distinct types [5, 6]:

- *Type I NETs* are associated with hypergastrinemia resulting from autoimmune atrophic gastritis; they are typically small (<1.0 cm), multiple, and multicentric. These tumors have an excellent clinical prognosis.
- *Type II NETs* occur in patients with multiple endocrine neoplasia type 1 and Zollinger-Ellison syndrome and are also associated with hypergastrinemia. Type II NETs are multiple and <1.5 cm.
- *Type III NETs* (sporadic) are not associated with hypergastrinemia. These tumors are generally solitary, arise in healthy gastric mucosa, and are not accompanied by ECL cell hyperplasia. Sporadic NETs progress to NEC (grade 3, mitotic count >20/HPF or Ki-67 index >20 %) and present with symptoms similar to those of gastric adenocarcinoma, often with distant metastases.

5.3.3   Small Intestine

Tumors of the small intestine are very rare. Microscopically these tumors resemble those in other parts of the gastrointestinal system. Most tumors are classified as adenocarcinomas, NETs, or GISTs [17].

Adenocarcinoma is predominantly found in patients with polyposis syndromes (familial adenomatous polyposis, MUTYH polyposis, Lynch syndrome, Peutz-Jeghers syndrome, and juvenile polyposis) and less frequently in patients with long-standing Crohn's disease. These tumors are graded using the 3-tiered system used for other adenocarcinomas [17].

Neuroendocrine tumors in the duodenum and the proximal jejunum usually measure less than 2.0 cm and may be multiple. These tumors are typically grade 1 and 2. NECs (grade 3) are larger

(2.0–4.0 cm) and may morphologically resemble small or large cell neuroendocrine carcinoma. In the distal jejunum and ileum, all neuroendocrine neoplasms reported to date are NETs (grade 1–2).

5.3.4 Ampulla of Vater

Malignant ampullary region tumors are either adenocarcinomas or neuroendocrine carcinomas. Adenocarcinomas are graded like homonymous tumors in other parts of the gastrointestinal system. The majority of ampullary neuroendocrine neoplasms (70 %) are NETs and 20 % are paragangliomas [18]. The remainder consists of NECs, which may show small cell and large cell differentiation. A significant portion of neuroendocrine carcinomas (>30 %) have an adenocarcinoma component and therefore are classified as MANECs.

5.3.5 Large Intestine

Tumors of the large intestine are the most common neoplasms of the gastrointestinal system. These tumors are usually adenocarcinomas, neuroendocrine neoplasms, or GISTs [19].

Adenocarcinomas of the large intestine are graded according to the previously described scheme (Fig. 5.4). In addition to the three conventional categories of differentiation (well, moderate, and poorly), the most recent WHO classification also includes the category of undifferentiated carcinoma (grade 4), characterized by complete lack of morphological, immunohistochemical, or molecular evidence of differentiation [19]. However, we believe, as do others, that while the designation of undifferentiated carcinoma is sensible, equating it to grade 4 adenocarcinoma is inappropriate since at the very core of its definition lays the absence of recognizable glandular structures. Hence, the morphology of these tumors provides no support for their inclusion into the category of adenocarcinomas.

The following variants of colonic adenocarcinoma are considered poorly differentiated:

- *Mucinous adenocarcinoma.* In this form of adenocarcinoma, more than 50 % of the tumor is composed of pools of extracellular mucin.
- *Signet ring cell carcinoma.* In order to classify a tumor into this category, over half of the tumor must be composed of signet ring cells.
- *Medullary carcinoma.* These tumors are composed of well-circumscribed sheets of mitotically active cells with vesicular nuclei,

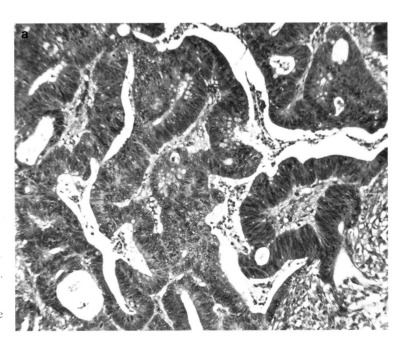

Fig. 5.4 Colonic adenocarcinoma. (**a**) Well-differentiated tumor with abundant glands displaying open lumina. (**b**) Moderately differentiated adenocarcinoma composed of both glandular and solid areas. (**c**) Poorly differentiated carcinoma arranged in solid sheets with only focal abortive glands

Fig. 5.4 (continued)

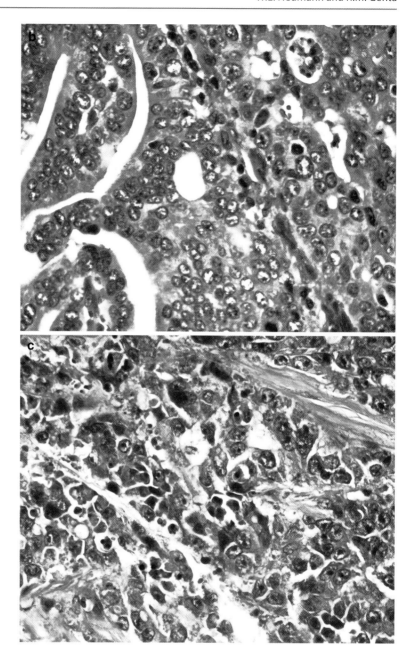

prominent nucleoli, abundant eosinophilic cytoplasm, and a marked lymphocytic infiltrate.

The mucinous, signet ring cell, and medullary subtypes may be associated with microsatellite instability and are usually less aggressive than their microsatellite stable counterparts.

5.3.6   Pancreas

Adenocarcinoma is the most common malignant tumor of the pancreas, and most of these arise from the pancreatic ducts and thus represent ductal adenocarcinomas [20]. The current grading system for ductal adenocarcinoma (Klöppel's

Fig. 5.5 Pancreatic adenocarcinoma. This moderately differentiated tumor exhibits moderate nuclear pleomorphism, irregular mucin production, and anastomosing glands correlating to a Klöppel grade 2

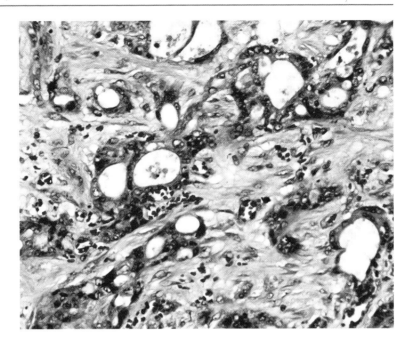

Table 5.2 Klöppel grading system for pancreatic adenocarcinoma adopted by WHO

Tumor grade	Glandular differentiation	Mucin production	Mitoses (per 10 HPF)	Nuclear features
Grade 1	Well differentiated	Intense	5	Little polymorphism, polar arrangement
Grade 2	Moderately differentiated duct-like structures and tubular glands	Irregular	6–10	Moderate pleomorphism
Grade 3	Poorly differentiated glands, abortive mucoepidermoid, and pleomorphic structures	Abortive	>10	Marked polymorphism and increased size

Source: Bosman FT, Carneiro F, Hruban RH, Theise ND (eds) (2010) World Health Organization classification of tumours. WHO classification of tumours of the digestive system, 4th edn. IARC Press, Lyon
HPF high-power field

grading scheme, endorsed and modified by the WHO) involves evaluation of gland-tubule formation, mucin production, mitotic count, and nuclear atypia (Fig. 5.5). Table 5.2 summarizes the 2010 WHO grading system of pancreatic adenocarcinomas [20].

5.3.7 Liver

Hepatocellular carcinoma (HCC) is most often of the classical type in which the cells retain some resemblance to normal liver cells [21]. Several other microscopic subtypes have been recognized including the following: fibrolamellar, scirrhous, undifferentiated, lymphoepithelioma like, and sarcomatoid [22].

HCC may be classified as well differentiated, moderately differentiated, and poorly differentiated (Fig. 5.6):

- *Well-differentiated hepatocellular carcinoma.* Most common in tumors less than 2.0 cm and rare in larger tumors. Neoplastic cells show minimal cytologic atypia with thin trabecular structures and pseudoglandular structures. Fatty change is frequent.
- *Moderately differentiated hepatocellular carcinoma.* Most common grade of HCC seen usually

in lesions greater than 3.0 cm. The tumoral cells have abundant eosinophilic cytoplasm and round nuclei with distinct nucleoli. Trabeculae are often greater than three cells thick. Pseudoglandular structures are common and often contain bile or proteinaceous material.

• *Poorly differentiated hepatocellular carcinoma*. This form of HCC grows in a solid pattern with slit-like vessels and loss of sinusoidal spaces. The tumor cells are pleomorphic with an increased nuclear-cytoplasmic ratio.

The WHO also recognizes an undifferentiated grade for hepatocellular carcinoma, which may be found in the central region of more differentiated tumors.

Cholangiocarcinoma is a relatively rare tumor in the USA but occurs more often in parts

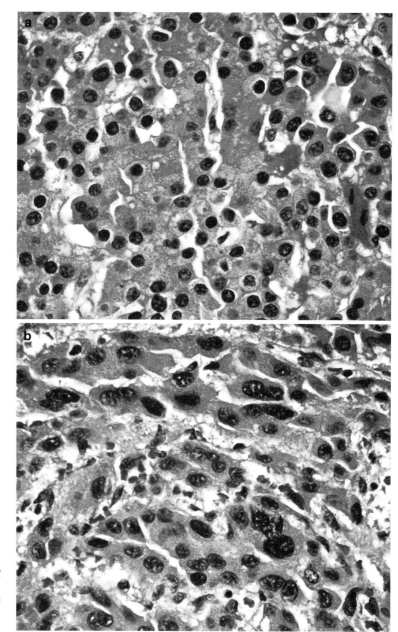

Fig. 5.6 Hepatocellular carcinoma (HCC). (**a**) Well-differentiated HCC with mildly hyperchromatic and irregular nuclei and an architecture with minimally thickened plates which may be difficult to distinguish from nonneoplastic liver. (**b**) Moderately differentiated HCC composed of cords of cells with pleomorphic and hyperchromatic nuclei. (**c**) Poorly differentiated HCC consisting of solid sheets of cells with crowded nuclei and little resemblance to normal liver

Fig. 5.6 (continued)

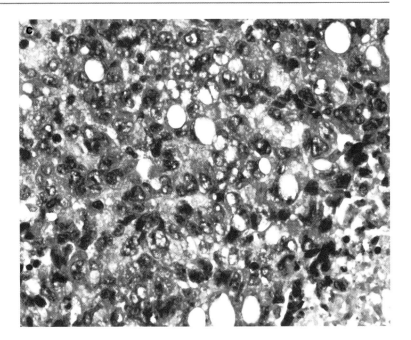

of Asia [23, 24]. According to the WHO [24], these tumors may be graded as well, moderately, or poorly differentiated depending on the extent of gland formation and the degree of cytological and architectural abnormalities (Fig. 5.7):

- *Well differentiated*. These tumors are composed of cuboidal cells that form uniform glands and papillary structures. Tumor cells may contain mucin, may be oncocytic, or can display squamous differentiation. The stroma is usually well developed, but some tumors may be highly desmoplastic.
- *Moderately differentiated*. These tumors form irregular glands, cribriform duct-like structures, cords, and solid nests. Desmoplastic stroma may be abundant.

- *Poorly differentiated*. These tumors are composed of pleomorphic cells with hyperchromatic nuclei arranged into solid sheets, strands, and nests. Gland formation may be focal. Some tumors are sarcomatoid and the spindled neoplastic cells may merge imperceptibly with the stroma. In some cases, the associated desmoplastic reaction may even render the malignant cells difficult to identify on routine H&E sections.

5.3.8   Gallbladder

Adenocarcinomas of the gallbladder may be graded as well, moderately, or poorly differentiated. These tumors are graded like the intrahepatic cholangiocarcinomas.

Fig. 5.7 Cholangiocarcinoma.
(**a**) Cuboidal cells line
numerous irregular glands
populating a desmoplastic
stroma in this well-differentiated tumor. (**b**) The solid
sheets and cords of this poorly
differentiated cholangiocarcinoma display only focal gland
formation

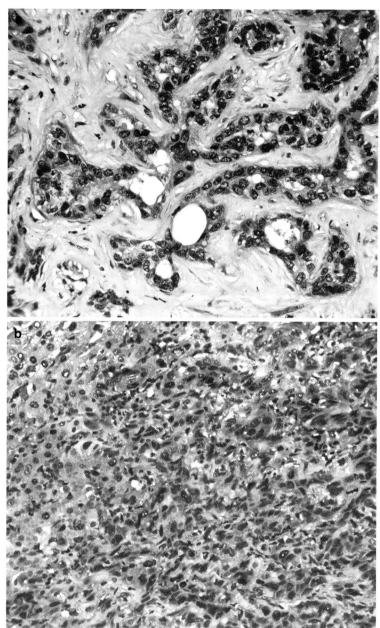

Books and Monographs

Bosman FT, Carneiro F, Hruban RH, Theise ND (eds)
(2010) World Health Organization classification of
tumours. WHO classification of tumours of the digestive system, 4th edn. IARC Press, Lyon

Iacobuzio-Donahue CA, Montgomery E, Goldblum JR
(eds) (2012) Gastrointestinal and liver pathology, foun-
dations in diagnostic pathology, 2nd edn. Elsevier
Saunders, Philadelphia

Odze RD, Goldblum JR (eds) (2009) Surgical pathology of
the GI tract, liver, biliary tract, and pancreas, 2nd edn.
Elsevier Saunders, Philadelphia

Articles

1. Montgomery E, Field JK, Boffetta P et al (2010)
World Health Organization classification of tumours.
WHO classification of tumours of the digestive system.

In: Bosman FT, Carneiro F, Hruban RH, Theise ND (eds) Squamous cell carcinoma of the oesophagus, 4th edn. IARC Press, Lyon, pp 18–24

2. Rindi G, Arnold R, Bosman FT et al (2010) Diagnostic terms revisited: nomenclature and classification of neuroendocrine neoplasms of the digestive system. In: Bosman FT, Carneiro F, Hruban RH, Theise ND (eds) World Health Organization classification of tumours. WHO classification of tumours of the digestive system, 4th edn. IARC Press, Lyon, pp 13–14

3. Rindi G, Kloppel G, Alhman H et al (2006) TNM staging of foregut (neuro)endocrine tumors: a consensus proposal including a grading system. Virchows Arch 449:395–401

4. Rindi G, Kloppel G, Couvelard A et al (2007) TNM staging of midgut and hindgut (neuro) endocrine tumors: a consensus proposal including a grading system. Virchows Arch 451:757–762

5. Rindi G, Bordi C, La Rosa S, Solcia E et al (2011) Gastroenteropancreatic (neuro)endocrine neoplasms: the histology report. Dig Liver Dis 43(Suppl 4):S356–S360

6. La Rosa S, Inzani F, Vanoli A et al (2011) Histologic characterization and improved prognostic evaluation of 209 gastric neuroendocrine neoplasms. Hum Pathol 42:1373–1384

7. Miettinen M, El-Rifai W, Sobin HL, Lasota J (2002) Evaluation of malignancy and prognosis of gastrointestinal stromal tumors: a review. Hum Pathol 33:478–483

8. Miettinen M, Sobin LH, Lasota J (2005) Gastrointestinal stromal tumors of the stomach: a clinicopathologic, immunohistochemical, and molecular genetic study of 1765 cases with long-term follow-up. Am J Surg Pathol 29:52–68

9. Miettinen M, Makhlouf H, Sobin LH, Lasota J (2006) Gastrointestinal stromal tumors of the jejunum and ileum: a clinicopathologic, immunohistochemical, and molecular genetic study of 906 cases before imatinib with long-term follow-up. Am J Surg Pathol 30:477–489

10. Miettinen M, Lasota J (2006) Gastrointestinal stromal tumors: review on morphology, molecular pathology, prognosis, and differential diagnosis. Arch Pathol Lab Med 130:1466–1478

11. Goh BK, Chow PK, Yap WM et al (2008) Which is the optimal risk stratification system for surgically treated localized primary GIST? Comparison of three contemporary prognostic criteria in 171 tumors and a proposal for a modified Armed Forces Institute of Pathology risk criteria. Ann Surg Oncol 15:2153–2163

12. Foo WC, Liegl-Atzwanger B, Lazar AJ (2012) Pathology of gastrointestinal stromal tumors. Clin Med Insights Pathol 5:23–33

13. Blay JY, Le Cesne A, Cassier PA, Ray-Coquard IL (2012) Gastrointestinal stromal tumors (GIST): a rare entity, a tumor model for personalized therapy, and yet ten different molecular subtypes. Discov Med 13:357–367

14. von Mehren M, Benjamin RS, Bui MM et al (2012) Soft tissue sarcoma, version 2.2012: featured updates to the NCCN guidelines. J Natl Compr Canc Netw 10:951–960

15. Huang Q, Shi J, Sun Q et al (2012) Distal esophageal carcinomas in Chinese patients vary widely in histopathology, but adenocarcinomas remain rare. Hum Pathol 43:2138–48

16. Lauwers GY, Carneiro F, Graham DY et al (2010) Tumors of the Stomach. In: Bosman FT, Carneiro F, Hruban RH, Theise ND (eds) World Health Organization classification of tumours. WHO classification of tumours of the digestive system, 4th edn. IARC, Lyon, pp 48–58

17. Shepherd NA, Carr NJ, Howe JR et al (2010) Tumours of the small intestine: carcinoma of the small intestine. In: Bosman FT, Carneiro F, Hruban RH, Theise ND (eds) World Health Organization classification of tumours. WHO classification of tumours of the digestive system, 4th edn. IARC Press, Lyon, pp 98–101

18. Garbrecht N, Anlauf M, Schmitt A et al (2008) Somatostatin-producing neuroendocrine tumors of the duodenum and pancreas: incidence, types, biological behavior, association with inherited syndromes, and functional activity. Endocr Relat Cancer 15:229–241

19. Hamilton SR, Bosman FT, Boffetta P et al (2010) Tumors of the colon and rectum: carcinoma of the colon and rectum. In: Bosman FT, Carneiro F, Hruban RH, Theise ND (eds) World Health Organization classification of tumours. WHO classification of tumours of the digestive system, 4th edn. IARC Press, Lyon, pp 134–146

20. Klöppel G, Lingenthal G, von Bülow M, Kern HF (1985) Histological and fine structural features of pancreatic ductal adenocarcinomas in relation to growth and prognosis: studies in xenografted tumours and clinico-histopathological correlation in a series of 75 cases. Histopathology 9:841–856

21. El-Serag HB (2011) Hepatocellular carcinoma. N Engl J Med 365:1118–1127

22. Theise ND, Curado MP, Franceschi S et al (2010) Tumors of the liver and intrahepatic bile ducts: hepatocellular carcinoma. In: Bosman FT, Carneiro F, Hruban RH, Theise ND (eds) World Health Organization classification of tumours. WHO classification of tumours of the digestive system, 4th edn. IARC Press, Lyon, pp 205–216

23. Tyson GL, El-Serag HB (2011) Risk factors for cholangiocarcinoma. Hepatology 54:173–184

24. Nakanuma Y, Curado MP, Franceschi S et al (2010) Tumors of the liver and intrahepatic bile ducts: intrahepatic cholangiocarcinoma. In: Bosman FT, Carneiro F, Hruban RH, Theise ND (eds) World Health Organization classification of tumours. WHO classification of tumours of the digestive system, 4th edn. IARC Press, Lyon, pp 217–2224

Endocrine System

6

Ivan Damjanov

6.1 Introduction

The grading of tumors of endocrine glands has been often difficult, inconsistent, and unrewarding. The reasons for these problems vary from one endocrine organ to another and from one tumor type to another, but in general, several explanations could be offered:

- The transition of hyperplasia to benign neoplasia to malignancy includes in many endocrine organs a spectrum of morphologic changes which are not always easily defined.
- The proposed grading systems are often complex and include a number of variants that are not acceptable to all pathologists. The lack of consensus among the pathologists has been one of the main hindrances to grading of most endocrine tumors.
- The correlation between the microscopic grading and the prognosis of tumors is often poor, and therefore, with a few notable exceptions, the clinicians do not find the pathologic grading of endocrine tumors to be as useful in the grading of tumors of some other organs systems.

I. Damjanov, M.D., Ph.D.
Department of Pathology,
The University of Kansas School of Medicine,
Kansas City, KS, USA
e-mail: idamjano@kumc.edu

6.2 Pituitary Tumors

Most pituitary tumors are classified as adenomas, which are further subtyped as hormonally active or inactive. Hormonally active adenomas are further classified on the basis of laboratory and immunohistochemical data as prolactinomas, growth hormone-secreting adenomas, corticotrophic adenomas, gonadotrophic adenomas, thyrotrophic adenomas, and plurihormonal mixed tumors. Standardized protocols have been developed for the handling and pathologic processing and reporting of pituitary tumors [1].

Small tumors measuring less than 10 mm in diameter are called microadenomas, whereas those that exceed 10 mm in diameter are called macroadenomas. Some of the macroadenomas have an aggressive growth and tend to recur after surgical resection. Pituitary carcinomas with extracranial metastases are extremely rare [2].

Microscopic grading of pituitary tumors is of limited clinical value because one cannot predict which tumors will be aggressive and recur after surgical resection and which one will be cured by initial surgery.

6.2.1 Comments

1. The aggressiveness of pituitary adenomas cannot be predicted from their histologic appearance. Thus, one can disregard the following microscopic findings:

- Areas of necrosis
- Bizarre enlarged nuclei
- Ring or giant nuclei
- Prominent nucleoli
- Mitotic figures

2. Prognostic indicators have been recently reviewed by Suhardja et al. [3]. The use of modern techniques such as DNA flow cytometry has been found to be of no clinical predictive value in assessing the invasiveness or persistence/recurrence of pituitary tumors.

6.3 Thyroid Tumors

Thyroid tumors are classified as benign or malignant. Thyroid adenomas outnumber carcinomas, which account for less than 1 % of all thyroid neoplasms.

Thyroid carcinomas are heterogeneous group tumors that occur in many histologic forms. Papillary carcinoma accounts for approximately 80 % of all carcinomas, forming with follicular carcinoma, medullary carcinoma, and undifferentiated (anaplastic) carcinomas, the vast majority of all thyroid tumors seen in general surgical pathology practice. The grading of thyroid tumors is of relative limited clinical significance [4, 5].

6.3.1 Comments

1. Papillary carcinoma of the thyroid may be graded microscopically. However, this grading system has not been widely used, and the recent reviews of the prognostic factors indicate that the size of the tumor and TNM staging are still the best predictors of tumor recurrence or resistance to therapy [6–9].

2. Follicular carcinoma cannot be graded adequately, but insular component, poorly differentiated carcinoma, trabecular component, serum thyroglobulin level before surgery, patient age at the time of presentation, solid component, and vascular invasion have adverse prognostic implications [10, 11]. The search for insular components seems to be warranted, since this pattern of growth has proven to be an independent risk factor. Hürthle cell pattern has also an adverse prognosis. The extent of necrosis and the proliferation index may also have prognostic value [11]. The significance or newly introduced terms such as follicular tumor of uncertain malignant potential, well-differentiated tumor of uncertain malignant potential, and well-differentiated carcinoma not otherwise specified remain to be determined in clinical-pathologic studies with long-term outcome [5].

Medullary carcinoma cannot be reliably graded. Nevertheless it has been noticed that certain microscopic findings correlate well with the aggressiveness of the tumors [12]. These microscopic findings include the following:
- High mitotic activity
- Foci of necrosis
- Small cell type
- Squamous differentiation

The prognosis is adversely affected by the finding of intravascular invasion, perineural invasion, extrathyroidal extension, and lymph node metastases [13]. The use of molecular biology and other probes has not contributed significantly to predicting the outcome of treatment [13, 14].

3. Undifferentiated carcinoma has an overall poor prognosis. Patients' advanced age, presence of necrosis (either focal or extensive), and mitotic count of more than three per ten high-power fields are associated with the worst outcome [15].

6.4 Parathyroid Tumors

Most of the parathyroid tumors are benign; parathyroid carcinomas are rare and may occur in both the usual location and ectopically [16, 17]. Microscopic grading of parathyroid tumors is not warranted, but the pathologist may be asked to contribute to the clinical-pathologic effort aimed at distinguishing parathyroid adenoma from parathyroid carcinoma.

6.4.1 Comments

1. Parathyroid adenomas often contain cells with enlarged hyperchromatic nuclei. These nuclear changes are not signs of malignancy [18].

2. The clinical and pathologic features favoring the diagnosis of parathyroid carcinoma are as follows:
   - Large size of the tumor
   - Adhesion of a hard tumor to adjacent structures
   - Extremely high serum levels of calcium and parathyroid hormone
   - Persistence of hyperparathyroidism after surgery
   - Microscopic invasion of the capsule and adjacent tissues
   - Vascular invasion
   - Fibrous bands subdividing the tumor into segments
   - Spindle-shaped nuclei of tumor cells
   - Mitotic activity
   - High labeling with MIB-1 antibodies
3. Many parathyroid tumors thought to be malignant do not recur, and better criteria distinguishing aggressive from nonaggressive parathyroid tumors need to be developed [17, 18].

6.5 Adrenal Cortical Tumors

Adrenal cortical tumors can be benign or malignant and hormonally active or inactive [19–21]. Most adrenocortical tumors are benign and are thus classified as adenomas; adrenocortical carcinomas are rare with an incidence of 0.5–2.0 cases per million population.

The grading of malignancy of adrenal cortical carcinomas is not routinely performed. Microscopic analysis is however useful for distinguishing these malignant tumors from benign adenomas.

6.5.1 Comments

1. The distinction of adrenocortical adenomas from carcinomas is not always simple. The size of the tumors is important: Tumors weighing more than 50 g and measuring 5 cm or more in greatest diameter are most likely malignant, whereas those that weigh less and are smaller are usually benign.
2. Several microscopic systems have been proposed to make the distinction more precise.

Four most widely used systems were recently reviewed by Lau and Weiss [19]. Here, we present only the system developed by Weiss because it is the simplest and thus the easiest to use in practice.

3. The Weiss system for diagnosing adrenal cortical carcinoma and separating it from adrenal cortical adenoma requires finding at least three criteria from the following list:
   - High nuclear grade
   - Mitotic rate exceeding five mitoses per 50 high-power fields
   - Atypical mitoses
   - Cells with clear cytoplasm accounting for more than 25 % of all cells
   - Diffuse growth pattern in more than 30 % of the tumor
   - Necrosis
   - Invasion into the veins
   - Invasion into the sinusoids
   - Invasion into the capsule

The nuclei are graded according to the system developed by Fuhrman for renal carcinoma, and "high nuclear grade" corresponds to Fuhrman grades 3 and 4. Aubert et al. [20] applied this system to their own material and found a correlation with clinical outcome in 98 % of the cases. The same authors reported that the immunohistochemical staining with MIB-1 may also help in predicting the malignancy of adrenocortical tumors. Giordano is also advocating the use of mitotic count for grading and formulating the prognosis for adrenocortical carcinoma [21]. Molecular biology with transcriptome profiling based on the study of ten genes may provide additional data that are of prognostic significance [22]. Nevertheless many challenging questions remain unanswered [23].

6.6 Adrenal Medullary Tumors

Adrenal medullary tumors comprise two groups: peripheral neuroblastic tumors (pNT), including neuroblastoma, ganglioneuroblastoma, and ganglioneuroma, and pheochromocytomas, i.e., tumors composed of chromaffin cells resembling adult medullary adrenal cells. Grading is an important part of the pathologic work-up of peripheral neuro-blastic tumors. Pheochromocytomas are not graded microscopically; however, microscopic study of these tumors may help in distinguishing those that are benign from those that are malignant.

6.7 Peripheral Neuroblastic Tumors

Neuroblastoma, ganglioneuroblastoma, and ganglioneuroma are tumors derived from immature sympathetic neuroblasts [24, 25]. Neuroblastomas occur most often in the adrenals of infants and children and less commonly in the extra-adrenal locations of the abdomen and the thoracic cavity. Ganglioneuroblastomas and ganglioneuromas also can occur in the adrenals but are more often found in extra-adrenal sites.

For practical purposes, these tumors are grouped under the heading of peripheral neuro-blastic tumors (pNT) and stratified according to the criteria of the International Neuroblastoma Pathology Classification (INPC). The INPC is based on the system developed by Shimada et al. [24] in 1984 and revised subsequently to incorporate molecular/genetic indicators [25–30].

On the basis of clinical, pathologic, and genetic/molecular findings, pNT are classified as tumors with favorable indicators and tumors with unfavorable indicators (Table 6.1). By combining these five indicators, the patients can be subdivided into three groups: low-risk, intermediate-risk, and high-risk groups [24, 25].

The microscopic grading system is based on the analysis of differentiation of tumor cells into Schwann cell-rich stroma and by estimating the proliferative capacity of tumor cells by calculating the so-called mitosis-karyorrhexis index (MKI).

The first step in the classification includes gross examination of tumors for the presence of nodules and a microscopic examination to determine the extent of schwannian differentiation. According to the degree of schwannian differentiation, pNT can be subdivided into two major groups (Fig. 6.1): tumors that contain less than 50 % of schwannian stroma (called "schwannian stroma poor" ["stroma poor"]), corresponding to neuroblastomas, and those with more than 50 % of schwannian stroma (called "schwannian stroma rich or dominant" ["stroma rich"]), ganglioneuromas, and ganglioneuroblastomas.

6.7.1 Stroma-Rich Peripheral Neuroblastic Tumors

The second step for evaluating schwannian stroma-poor pNT (neuroblastomas) is to analyze them microscopically and classify into three groups, i.e., as undifferentiated, poorly differentiated, and differentiating neuroblastoma (Fig. 6.2):

- *Neuroblastoma undifferentiated.* These tumors are composed of undifferentiated cells, whose neuroblastic nature can be definitely proven only by additional immunohistochemical or ultra-structural studies. These neuroblasts have small-to-medium size nuclei surrounded with scant cytoplasm that has indistinct borders. The nuclei contain finely granular or stippled ("salt and pepper"-like) chromatin and occasional nucleoli. Between the cells, there is no discernible neuro-pil. Foci of necrosis, exudates of fibrin, or collagenous stroma may be seen but should not be mistaken for schwannian differentiation.
- *Neuroblastoma, poorly differentiated.* These tumors are composed of undifferentiated neuro-blasts but also contain streaks of neuropil

Table 6.1 Classification of peripheral neuroblastic tumors according to the prognostic parameters

Parameter	Favorable	Unfavorable
Age at diagnosis	Less than 1 year	1 year or more
Clinical stage	Stage 1 or 2 or 4S	Stage 3 or 4
Histopathology	Favorable	Unfavorable
MYCN oncogene	Non-amplified	Amplified
DNA ploidy	Hyperdiploid	Diploid
Urinary catecholamines	Elevated	Low

Source: Modified from tables in Wenig et al. (1997) and Shimada et al. [24–26]

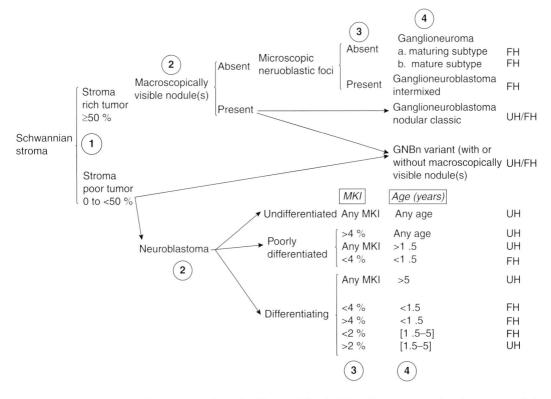

Fig. 6.1 International neuroblastoma pathology classification. The circled numbers correspond to the recommended steps described in the text. Based on diagrams in the papers of Shimada et al. [24–26] and Peuchmaur et al. [27]

corresponding to focal schwannian differentiation. Up to 5 % of all tumor cells differentiate into ganglion cells. These ganglion cells must be distinguished from neuroblasts that have pleomorphic and anaplastic or bizarre nuclei and multiple nucleoli. The extent of neuropil formation varies from one tumor to another but also from one section of the same tumor to another.

- *Neuroblastoma, differentiating.* These tumors are composed of neuroblastic cells that show focal neuronal differentiation. Differentiating neuroblasts and ganglion cells account for 5 % or more of all tumor cells. Differentiating neuroblasts show synchronous enlargement of nuclei and cytoplasm. The vesicular nucleus of these cells is located eccentrically in a well-developed cytoplasm, which appears eosinophilic or amphophilic and has clear-cut cell borders. Mature ganglion cells may be seen as well.
- The extent of schwannian stroma formation varies, but by definition, stroma comprises

less than 50 % of the entire tumor. The amount of schwannian neuropil is not critical for distinguishing poorly differentiated from differentiating neuroblastoma. It is usually most prominent at the periphery of tumor nests but does not lead to the formation of nodules or distinct separation of the undifferentiated from the differentiated part of the tumor. The continuity between the stroma-poor and stroma-enriched parts of differentiating neuroblastoma is a very important feature of these tumors, allowing one to distinguish them from ganglioneuroblastoma nodular type.

The third step in evaluating the schwannian stroma-poor pNT includes counting of mitoses and karyorrhectic nuclei (mitosis-karyorrhexis index – MKI). Mitotic figures are recognized by their rod-shaped condensation of chromatin, spiked projections of chromatin, and a lack of nuclear membrane. Karyorrhexis leads to condensation of the chromatin and fragmentation of

Fig. 6.2 Peripheral neuroblastic tumors classified as
"schwannian stroma-poor
tumors." (**a**) Undifferentiated
tumor, composed almost
exclusively of densely
compacted neuroblastic cells.
(**b**) Poorly differentiated
tumor composed of immature
neuroblasts with focal streaks
of neuropil corresponding to
schwannian differentiation.
(**c**) Differentiating neuroblastoma consists of undifferentiated and differentiating
neuroblastic cells and a
well-developed neuropil

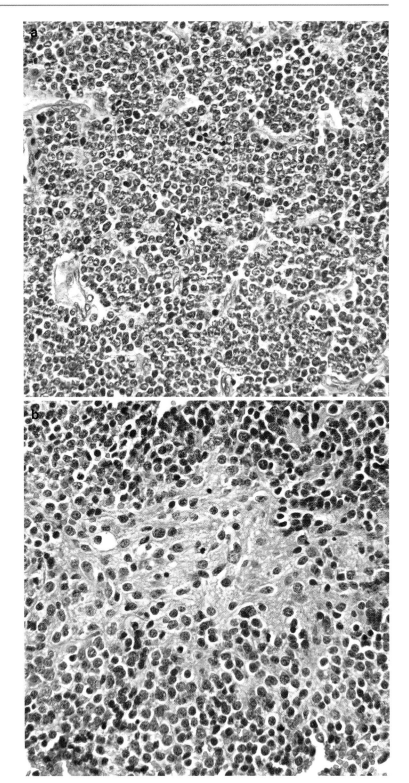

Fig. 6.2 (continued)

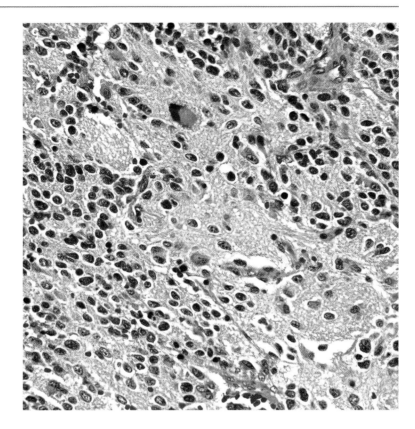

nuclear material, accompanied by eosinophilic condensation of the cytoplasm. It is necessary to count 5,000 cells and then express the MKI as low, 2 % (<100/5,000); intermediate, 2–4 % (100–200/5,000); or high, >4 % (>200/5,000).

The fourth step involves inclusion of clinical data, primarily the age of the patient. Using the guidelines outlined in Fig. 6.1, the histologic findings are then classified as favorable histology (FH) or unfavorable histology (UH).

6.7.2   Stroma-Rich Tumors

The second step for tumors that contain more than 50 % of schwannian stroma (*stroma-rich tumors*) involves evaluation for nodularity. Nodules may be visible on gross examination or only microscopically.

The third step for evaluating the tumors that show no nodularity includes a microscopic examination to determine whether the tumor contains

neuroblastic cells. If no neuroblastic foci are found, the tumor is classified as ganglioneuroma, maturing subtype. If microscopic neuroblastic cells are present, the tumor is classified as ganglioneuroblastoma, intermixed. Both of these tumors have favorable histology (FH).

If macroscopically visible nodule(s) are present, the tumor may be classified as ganglioneuroblastoma, nodular, classic, or ganglioneuroblastoma variant (GNBn). Some of the ganglioneuroblastoma variants have no macroscopically visible nodules but are associated with metastases that show neuroblastomatous features.

Principal features of stroma-rich tumor are illustrated in the Fig. 6.3 and briefly summarized as follows:

• *Ganglioneuroma.* This tumor is composed predominantly of ganglioneuromatous stroma. If it is composed of mature Schwann cells and ganglion cells, it is subclassified as *ganglioneuroma, mature subtype.* If it also contains foci of differentiating neuroblasts, it is subclassified as *ganglioneuroma,*

Fig. 6.3 Peripheral neuroblastic tumors classified as "schwannian stroma-rich tumors."
(**a**) Ganglioneuroma, mature, consists of ganglion cells and schwannian cells.
(**b**) Ganglioneuroma, maturing subtype, consists of maturing neuroblasts and ganglion cells in a schwannian stroma.
(**c**) Ganglioneuroblastoma, intermixed, is composed predominantly of ganglioneuromatous tissue forming more than 50 % of the entire tumor. However, it also contains residual microscopic neuroblastic foci, seen as small blue cells

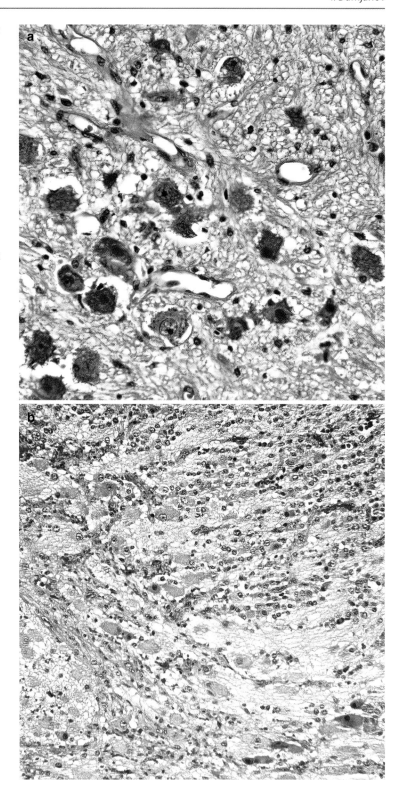

Fig. 6.3 (continued)

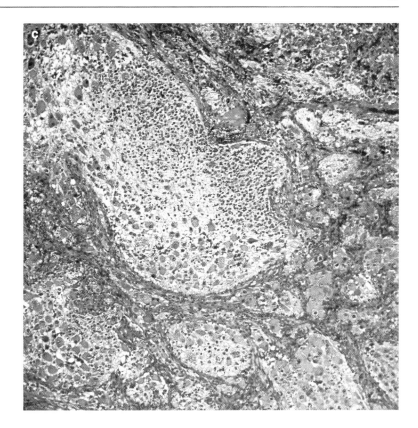

maturing subtype. Maturing neuroblastomatous cells are intermixed with schwannian cells and do not form distinct nests as in the intermixed from of ganglioneuroblastoma.

- *Ganglioneuroblastoma, intermixed.* This tumor is composed predominantly of ganglioneuromatous tissue forming more than 50 % of the entire tumor. However, it also contains residual microscopic neuroblastic foci. Because of these "residual neuroblasts," this tumor must be differentiated from ganglioneuroblastoma, nodular subtype, a tumor that contains hemorrhagic nodule or nodules composed of highly aggressive tumor cells.

- *Ganglioneuroblastoma, nodular.* Typically this tumor may present a single hemorrhagic nodule or in form of several hemorrhagic nodules surrounded by grayish-white tissue. Microscopically, it has a characteristic composite nature, containing both stroma-rich/stroma-dominant nodules and stroma-poor nodules. Thus, some nodules are composed of undifferentiated neuroblastic cells, whereas others have the features of ganglioneuroblastoma intermixed and ganglioneuroma.

- *Ganglioneuroblastoma variant.* These tumors can be nodular on gross examination or show no nodularity [26]. Some tumors are not nodular but have metastases. It should be noticed that some tumors in this category have more and some have less than 50 % of schwannian stroma. It has been shown that the nodules can be classified as favorable or unfavorable. The favorable nodules include poorly differentiating or differentiating and low or intermediate MKI tumors in children under the age of 1.5 year. The unfavorable nodules in children under 1.5 years of age are composed of undifferentiated cells and have a high MKI. In the age group between 1.5 and 5 years, the nodules are composed of undifferentiated tumors or poorly differentiated tumors with an intermediate or high MKI. In children over the age of 5 years, all tumors of this type are considered to have unfavorable histology.

6.7.3 Comments

1. The grading and prognostic stratification of peripheral neuroblastic tumors are constantly upgraded with data obtained by studies based on the application of cytogenetics, immunohistochemistry, and molecular biology [27, 28]. Ultimately this will lead to new revisions of the INPC criteria.

2. Excellent treatment results are obtained in asymptomatic low-risk neuroblastoma patients stages 2a and 2b [30].Older patients or those who have unfavorable histology tumors have a less favorable prognosis, but even so the risk stratification is not ideal and needs to be refined.

3. Pheochromocytomas are not graded routinely. Most pheochromocytomas are benign, but approximately 10 % are malignant [31]. Microscopic data are used for predicting the malignancy of these tumors, although this might be extremely difficult [32]. A scoring system for predicting the malignancy of pheochromocytoma has been proposed by Thompson [32]. The findings favoring the diagnosis of malignancy include the following:
   - Invasive growth:
     - Capsular invasion
     - Vascular invasion
     - Invasion of the periadrenal fat tissue
   - Architectural features:
     - "Large nests" exceeding three to four time the size of normal paraganglia
     - Diffuse growth of tumor cells
     - Increased cellularity with nuclear monotony
     - Central of confluent necrosis
   - Cellular and nuclear features:
     - Spindle-shaped or small cells
     - Cellular and nuclear pleomorphism
     - Nuclear hyperchromasia
     - Macronucleoli
   - Mitoses:
     - Increased activity (>3 per 10 hpf)
     - Atypical mitoses

4. Up to 30 % of all pheochromocytoma patients have germ line mutations involving one of the well-known tumor susceptibility genes, resulting in well-defined multiple tumor syndromes [33, 34]. Thus, pheochromocytomas develop as part of multiple endocrine neoplasia type 2 due to mutations in the RET gene, von Hippel-Lindau disease caused by mutation of VHL gene, hereditary paraganglioma syndromes resulting from mutations of succinate dehydrogenase genes (SDHD, SDHAF2, SDHC, SDHB), neurofibromatosis type 1 due to mutations of the NF1 gene, and familial pheochromocytoma syndromes due to mutations of the SDHA, TMEM127, and MAX genes. Genetic testing of pheochromocytoma patients is thus a high-yield procedure because it can identify patients at risk of relapse of pheochromocytoma or multiple pheochromocytomas.

6.8 Pancreatic Neuroendocrine Neoplasms

The participants of the North American Neuroendocrine Society on neuroendocrine tumor consensus conferences agreed that the pancreatic neuroendocrine tumors (NET) should be separated from neuroendocrine tumors of the stomach and intestines [35, 36]. According to the general consensus, NET are to be classified into three groups: low grade, intermediate grade, and high grade. However, no specific system of grading was recommended, and accordingly, new approaches are being developed to provide better grading of PEN [37]. In several clinical-pathologic studies, including a recent large international study on over 1,000 patients, it has been shown that microscopic grading has clinical and prognostic value, but it is not routinely practiced [38].

6.8.1 Comment

1. On the basis of microscopic findings alone, it is not possibly easy to predict which islet cell tumor will be clinically benign and which one will have a more aggressive growth and metastasize. The only exception is the small cell carcinomas that resemble small cell ("oat-cell") carcinomas of the lungs which are highly malignant and are readily identifiable microscopically.

2. Immunohistochemistry with antibodies to KIT (CD117) and cytokeratin CK19 can generate data that have prognostic significance [37].

Table 6.2 Mayo Clinic pancreatic endocrine tumors three-tiered grading system

Feature	Score
Mitoses	
0 per 50 hpf	0
1–3 per 50 hpf	1
4 or more per 50 hpf	2
Necrosis	
Absent	0
Present	1
Tumor border	
Noninfiltrating	0
Infiltrating	1
Total	0–4

Source: Based on the data in Zhang et al. [37]
Grade 1 tumors = score 0–1
Grade 2 tumors = score 2
Grade 3 tumors = score 3–4

Low-risk tumors are KIT−/CK19−, intermediate-risk tumors are KIT−/CK19+, and high-risk tumors are KIT+/CK19+ [37].

3. In a study of almost 100 pancreatic endocrine tumors, Mayo Clinic pathologists have found that the three groups of PEN differ one from another with regard to the following parameters: tumor size, mitoses, infiltrative borders, extrapancreatic extension, perineural invasion, and presence of amyloid [37]. To simplify the grading system, they have proposed to use only three variables: mitoses, necrosis, and infiltrating/noninfiltrating tumor borders. This three-tiered system correlates well with the KIT/CK19 system and is readily applicable in practice (Table 6.2). There was a significant difference in the survival, tumor metastasis, tumor recurrence, and functional activity of tumors in these three groups.

Books and Monographs

DeLellis RA, Lloyd RV, Heitz PU, Eng C (eds) (2004) World Health Organization classification of tumours. Pathology and genetics. Tumours of endocrine organs. IARC Press, Lyon

Solcia E, Capella C, Klöppel G (1997) Tumors of the pancreas. Atlas of tumor pathology, 3rd series, Fascicle 20. Armed Forces Institute of Pathology, Washington, DC

Wenig BM, Heffess CS, Adair CF (1997) Atlas of endocrine pathology. W.B. Saunders, Philadelphia

Articles

1. Nose V, Ezzat S, Horvath E et al (2011) Protocol for the examination of specimens from patients with primary pituitary tumors. Arch Pathol Lab Med 135:640–646
2. Lamas C, Nunez R, Garcia-Uria J et al (2004) Malignant prolactinoma with multiple bone and pulmonary metastases. Case report. J Neurosurg 101(1 Suppl):116–121
3. Suhardja A, Kovacs K, Greenberg O et al (2005) Prognostic indicators in pituitary tumors. Endocr Pathol 16:1–9
4. Akslen LA, LiVolsi VA (2000) Prognostic significance of histologic grading compared with subclassification of papillary thyroid carcinoma. Cancer 88:1902–1908
5. Sobrinho-Simões M, Eloy C, Magalhaes J et al (2011) Follicular thyroid carcinoma. Mod Pathol 24(Suppl 2): S10–S18
6. Leboulleux S, Rubino C, Baudin E et al (2005) Prognostic factors for persistent or recurrent disease of papillary thyroid carcinoma with neck lymph node metastases and/or tumor extension beyond the thyroid capsule at initial diagnosis. J Clin Endocrinol Metab 90:5723–5729
7. Baloch ZW, LiVolsi VA (2005) Pathologic diagnosis of papillary thyroid carcinoma: today and tomorrow. Expert Rev Mol Diagn 5:573–584
8. Siironen P, Louhimo J, Nordling S et al (2005) Prognostic factors in papillary thyroid cancer: an evaluation of 601 consecutive patients. Tumour Biol 26:57–64
9. Machens A, Holzhausen HJ, Dralle H (2005) The prognostic value of primary tumor size in papillary and follicular thyroid carcinoma. Cancer 103:2269–2273
10. Yamashita H, Noguchi Y, Noguchi S et al (2005) Significance of an insular component in follicular thyroid carcinoma with distant metastasis at initial presentation. Endocr Pathol 16:41–48
11. Ghossein R (2009) Problems and controversies in the histopathology of thyroid carcinomas of follicular cell origin. Arch Pathol Lab Med 133:683–691
12. Franc B, Rosenberg-Bourgin M, Caillou B et al (1998) Medullary thyroid carcinoma: search for histological predictors of survival (109 prob and cases analysis). Hum Pathol 29:1078–1084
13. Clark JR, Fridman TR, Odell MJ et al (2005) Prognostic variables and calcitonin in medullary thyroid cancer. Laryngoscope 115:1445–1450
14. Leboulleux S, Baudin E, Travagli JP, Schlumberger M (2004) Medullary thyroid carcinoma. Clin Endocrinol (Oxf) 61:299–310
15. Volante M, Cavallo GP, Papotti M (2004) Prognostic factors of clinical interest in poorly differentiated carcinomas of the thyroid. Endocr Pathol 15:313–317
16. Moran CA, Suster S (2005) Primary parathyroid tumors of the mediastinum: a clinicopathologic and immunohistochemical study of 17 cases. Am J Clin Pathol 124:749–754
17. Wei CH, Harari A (2012) Parathyroid carcinoma: update and guidelines for management. Curr Treat Options Oncol 13:11–23
18. Kameyama K, Takami H (2005) Proposal for the histological classification of parathyroid carcinoma. Endocr Pathol 16:49–52

19. Lau SK, Weiss LM (2005) Adrenocortical neoplasms. Pathol Case Reviews 10:219–228

20. Aubert S, Wacrenier A, Leroy X et al (2002) Weiss system revisited: a clinicopathologic and immunohistochemical study of 49 adrenocortical tumors. Am J Surg Pathol 26:1612–1619

21. Giordano TJ (2011) The argument for mitotic rate-based grading for the prognostication of adrenocortical carcinoma. Am J Surg Pathol 35:471–473

22. Giordano TJ (2010) Adrenocortical tumors: an integrated clinical, pathologic, and molecular approach at the University of Michigan. Arch Pathol Lab Med 134:1440–1443

23. Lehmann T, Wrzesinski T (2012) The molecular basis of adrenocortical cancer. Cancer Genet 205: 131–137

24. Shimada H, Bonadio J, Sano H (2005) Neuroblastoma and related tumors. Pathol Case Rev 10:252–256

25. Shimada H, Chatten J, Newton WA et al (1984) Histopathologic prognostic factors in neuroblastic tumors: definition of subtypes of ganlioneuroblastoma and age-linked classification of neuroblastomas. J Natl Cancer Inst 73:405–416

26. Shimada H, Ambros IM, Dehner LP et al (1999) The International Neuroblastoma Pathology Classification the Shimada system. Cancer 86:364–372

27. Peuchmaur M, d'Amore ESG, Joshi VV et al (2003) Revision of International Neuroblastoma Pathology Classification: confirmation of favorable and unfavorable prognostic subsets in ganglioneuroblastoma, nodular. Cancer 98:2274–2281

28. Weinstein JL, Katzenstein HM, Cohn SL (2003) Advances in the diagnosis and treatment of neuroblastoma. Oncologist 8:278–292

29. Attiyeh EF, London WB, Mosse YP, Children's Oncology Group et al (2005) Chromosome 1p and 11q deletions and outcome in neuroblastoma. N Engl J Med 353:2243–2253

30. Strother DR, London WB, Schmidt ML et al (2012) Outcome after surgery or with restricted use of chemotherapy for patients with low-risk neuroblastoma: results of Children's Oncology Group study P9641. J Clin Oncol 30:1842–1848

31. Thompson LDR (2005) Pheochromocytoma. Pathol Case Rev 10:243–251

32. Thompson LDR (2002) Pheochromocytoma of the adrenal gland scaled score (PASS) to separate benign from malignant neoplasms: a clinicopathologic and immunophenotypic study of 100 cases. Am J Surg Pathol 26:551–566

33. Bausch B, Malinoc A, Maruscke L et al (2012) Genetics of pheochromocytoma. Chirurg 83: 511–518

34. Cascon A, Robledo M (2012) MAX and MYC: a heritable breakup. Cancer Res 72:3119–3124

35. Klimstra DS, Adsay NV, Chetty R et al (2010) Pathology reporting of neuroendocrine tumors: application of the Delphic consensus process to the development of a minimum pathology data set. Am J Surg Pathol 34:300–313

36. Klimstra DS, Modlin IR, Coppola D et al (2010) The pathologic classification of neuroendocrine tumors: review of nomenclature, grading and staging systems. Pancreas 39:707–712

37. Zhang L, Lohse CM, Dao LN, Smyrk TC (2011) Proposed histopathologic grading system derived from a study of KIT and CK19 expression in pancreatic endocrine neoplasm. Hum Pathol 42:324–331

38. Rindi G, Falconi M, Klersy C et al (2012) TNM staging of neoplasms of the endocrine pancreas: results from a large international cohort study. J Natl Cancer Inst 104:764–777

Tumors of the Kidney

7

Ivan Damjanov

Tumors of the kidneys form a rather heterogeneous group of neoplasms. Malignant tumors predominate, and among these, clear cell renal cell carcinoma accounts for most of the neoplasms. Papillary renal cell carcinoma comprises approximately 10–15 %, chromophobe 5 %, and carcinoma of the collecting duct of Bellini less than 1 % of all renal malignancies. Approximately 4–5 % of renal malignant tumors cannot be properly classified and are grouped under the heading of renal cell carcinoma unclassified. All other malignant renal tumors are rare (Eble et al. 2004; Murphy et al. 2004; Bostwick and Cheng 2008).

7.1 Clear Cell Renal Cell Carcinoma

As implied in its name, this most common renal tumor is composed of clear cells. The historical aspects and the controversies surrounding the grading of renal cell carcinomas have been comprehensively reviewed by Delahunt [1]. Tumor grade, together with positive surgical resection margins, presence of metastases, pTNM stage, tumor type, and sarcomatoid architecture, is considered to belong to the category 1 prognostic factors [2]. Even though there is no consensus on the merits and reproducibility of various grading systems, the grading system proposed by Fuhrman et al. [3] has been most widely used and tested and is included in the WHO text (Eble et al. 2004). This four-tiered system is presented here.

Fuhrman Grading System. The tissue is examined at low magnification, and the most anaplastic ("worst") area is identified for grading. The grading takes into account the size and shape of nuclei, the chromatin pattern, and the presence of nucleoli as follows:

- *Grade 1 tumors*. Tumor cells have uniform, round, small nuclei (<10 μm) comparable to the nuclei of lymphocytes. The chromatin is condensed, and the nucleoli are not visible (Fig. 7.1).
- *Grade 2 tumors*. Tumor cells have somewhat larger, round vesicular nuclei (15 μm), with finely dispersed chromatin. The nucleoli are not present or are not clearly visible at low magnification (Fig. 7.2).
- *Grade 3 tumors* have still larger nuclei (>20 μm), which are round or oval and contain finely dispersed chromatin. The nucleoli are easily seen at low magnification (Fig. 7.3).
- *Grade 4 tumors*. Tumor cells have irregularly shaped hyperchromatic large nuclei (>20 μm) that vary in size and shape. The chromatin is irregularly distributed, and the nucleoli are large ("macronucleoli") (Fig. 7.4).

I. Damjanov, M.D., Ph.D.
Department of Pathology, The University
of Kansas School of Medicine,
Kansas City, KS, USA
e-mail: idamjano@kumc.edu

I. Damjanov, F. Fan (eds.), *Cancer Grading Manual*,
DOI 10.1007/978-3-642-34516-6_7, © Springer-Verlag Berlin Heidelberg 2013

Fig. 7.1 Renal cell
carcinoma. Fuhrman grade 1
tumor has small condensed
nuclei

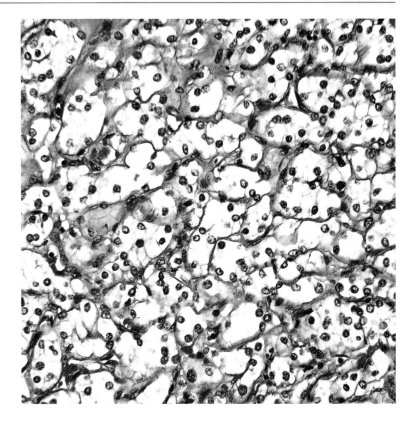

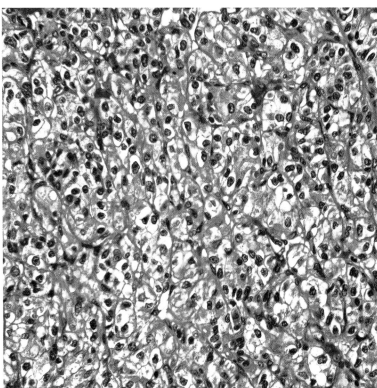

Fig. 7.2 Renal cell
carcinoma. Fuhrman grade 2
tumor has small vesicular
nuclei, which contain no
obvious nucleoli

Fig. 7.3 Renal cell carcinoma. Fuhrman grade 3 tumor has enlarged vesicular nuclei, which contain obvious nucleoli

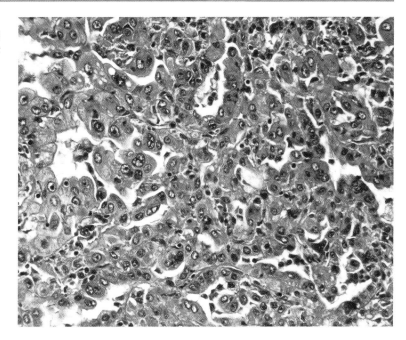

Fig. 7.4 Renal cell carcinoma. Fuhrman grade 4 tumor. The nuclei of this tumor show pleomorphism and appear hyperchromatic

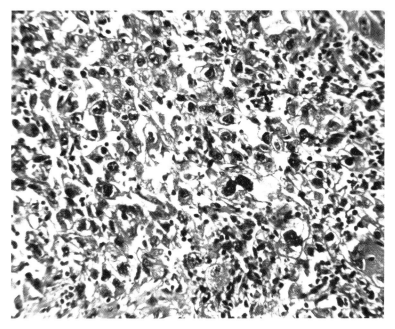

The details of the grading system are summarized in the Table 7.1.

7.1.1 Comments

1. Most RCC (>80 %) are classified as grade 2 or 3; grade 1 and 4 tumors are uncommon accounting for only 5–10 % of all cases.

2. Fuhrman grade has been shown to be an independent prognostic factor for the patients who have clear cell renal cell carcinomas [4–6].

3. Significant interobserver and intraobserver variability is a considerable drawback in using the Fuhrman grading system [1, 7]. This problem has prompted attempts to consolidate the four grade system into a more reproducible three- or

Table 7.1 Grading of renal cell carcinomas according to Fuhrman

Grade	Nuclear size (μm)	Nuclear shape	Chromatin pattern	Nucleoli
1	<10	Round, uniform	Condensed	Not evident
2	15	Round, uniform	Finely granular, dispersed	Rudimentary, not seen at low magnification[a]
3	20	Round or oval, slightly variable	Coarsely granular	Clearly visible at low magnification[a]
4	>20	Pleomorphic, multilobated	Hyperchromatic and clumped	Large ("macronucleoli")

Source: Modified from Murphy et al. (2004)

[a]We prefer to use the 20× objective rather than the 10× objective recommended in the above-listed reference; that way, we can much easier distinguish nucleoli from coarse condensations of chromatin in grade 2 tumors

two-tiered system [8] or to propose grading based on nucleolar prominence [9]. For the time being, Fuhrman grading system remains still the most widely used approach [10].

4. Renal cell carcinomas showing focally rhabdoid or sarcomatoid spindle-cell morphology grow aggressively and should be classified as high-grade tumors with a poor prognosis [1, 11, 12].

7.2 Papillary Renal Cell Carcinoma

Papillary renal cell carcinoma (PRCC) is the second most common histologic type of renal cell carcinoma in the surgical pathology material. Overall, it might be even the most common renal tumors since they are found in 23 % of adult autopsies [12]. Papillary renal tumors smaller than 5 mm are by convention classified as papillary adenomas.

Overall, PRCC has a better prognosis than clear cell renal cell carcinoma, but the significance of various prognostic parameters remains to be determined [12, 13]. According to Delahunt and Eble, papillary carcinomas can be divided into two subtypes [14]. *Type 1* tumors consist of papillae lines by a single layer of small cells with pale or basophilic cytoplasm and uniform small oval nuclei. *Type 2* tumors are composed of papillae covered by pseudostratified or multilayered epithelium comprising large cells with eosinophilic cytoplasm and large irregularly shaped nuclei. Histologic typing of papillary renal cell carcinoma has been found to have prognostic significance [14], although these differences seem to disappear if applied to tumors which have

spread beyond the confines of the kidney or those that have metastasized [15].

Grading of PRCC remains controversial. Some urologic pathologists feel that the Fuhrman system provides the best approach to grading of PRCC [16], whereas others think that Fuhrman system should not be used on PRCC [17]. Delahunt pointed out that neither nuclear size nor nuclear pleomorphism of PRCC correlates well with the clinical outcome of the malignant disease [1]. However, nucleolar prominence shows such correlation [17]. Accordingly, Delahunt and his associates recommend assessment of the nucleolar prominence under high-power magnification in areas of the tumor showing greatest pleomorphism and use it as the only reliable parameter for grading PRCC [1, 17].

7.3 Chromophobe Renal Cell Carcinoma

The grading of chromophobe renal cell carcinomas (CRRC) is controversial, especially since these tumors have a tendency to show considerable nuclear pleomorphism [18, 19]. Most authorities are opposed to using Fuhrman grading system on CRRC [20]. Others are advocating a modified three-tiered system [21]. Additional modifications of the three-tiered system have also been tested [22].

Cheville and his associates from Mayo Clinic reviewed a large number CRRC using the three-tiered chromophobe RCC grade of Paner et al. [21] and found that the grading did not add any prognostic information beyond what was already gained from the TNM stage grouping of tumors and the identification of sarcomatoid changes [23]. It thus appears that the grading of CRCC is not warranted. The presence of tumor necrosis and sarcomatoid change should be noted and quantitated, since these findings have prognostic significance [10].

7.4 Collecting Duct Carcinoma

Collecting duct carcinoma is a rare, highly aggressive malignant tumor accounting for less than 1 % of all renal malignancies. It is thought to originate from the principal cells of the collecting ducts of Bellini (Eble et al. 2004). Microscopically, the tumor is in essence an adenocarcinoma with tubular, tubulopapillary features, solid areas, and even sarcomatoid parts [24]. The tumor cells have high-grade nuclei, corresponding to Fuhrman grade 3 and 4 nuclei. Collecting duct carcinoma shows overlapping morphologic features with medullary carcinoma, another rare high-grade renal tumor [24].

7.5 Unclassified Renal Cell Carcinoma

Renal cell carcinomas that do not fit into any of the four well-known categories (clear cell, papillary, chromophobe, or collecting duct carcinoma) are assigned to the category of unclassified renal cell carcinomas. In the 2004 classification of renal tumors, the experts of the WHO have defined the following criteria for including renal tumors into this category: composites of recognized renal tumor subtypes, pure sarcomatoid morphology without recognizable epithelial elements, mucin production, rare admixture of malignant epithelial and stromal elements, and unrecognized cell types (Eble et al. 2004).

Unclassified renal cell carcinomas are obviously a heterogenous group of tumors [25]. Most tumors are usually diagnosed at an advances stage and have bad prognosis [25].Grading may contribute to the prognosis, but most tumors have high-grade nuclei [25].Other factors that have prognostic significance are tumor size, TNM stage, tumor coagulative necrosis, microvascular invasion, and pure sarcomatoid phenotype.

7.6 Urothelial Carcinoma Involving the Renal Pelvis

Urothelial tumors originating in the renal pelvis account for approximately 5–7 % of all renal neoplasms [26, 27]. In contrast to urothelial tumors of the lower urinary tract, these tumors are mostly high grade, typically diagnosed in a high stage. Most tumors of the renal pelvis are classified as urothelial carcinomas, but up to 40 % of them show unusual morphologic features. These unusual morphologic aspects include the following:
- Micropapillary carcinoma
- Lymphoepithelioma-like carcinoma
- Sarcomatoid carcinoma
- Squamous differentiation or overt squamous carcinoma
- Clear cell carcinoma
- Adenocarcinoma
- Rhabdoid carcinoma
- Signet-ring carcinoma
- Plasmacytoid carcinoma

Some tumors show pseudosarcomatous stromal changes, and some show intratubular extension into the renal parenchyma [26]. Urothelial carcinomas are graded the same way as those from the lower urinary tract. Most of the metaplastic and/or heterologous components have high-grade nuclei.

7.7 Rare Tumor Types

The clinical value of grading of rare renal tumors cannot be verified due to their uncommon occurrence and a lack of large series. Most of these tumors are thus by prevailing consensus classified as either high-grade or low-grade neoplasms:

Renal cell carcinoma associated with transcription factor E3 expression and Xp11.2 translocation. This uncommon tumor is by definition a high-grade neoplasm, characterized by a tendency for metastatic spread, which carries a poor prognosis [28].

Thyroid-like follicular carcinoma of the kidney. This rare tumor is a low-grade malignancy, although there are reports that it may metastasize [29, 30].

Mucinous tubular and spindle-cell carcinoma. This is a low-grade malignancy, and most tumors remain localized to the kidney [31, 32]. Occasionally, some tumors may contain obviously malignant spindle-cell areas, but some tumors have metastasized even without evidence of such a sarcomatoid component [33].

Books and Monographs

Bostwick DG, Cheng L (2008) Urologic surgical pathology, 2nd edn. Mosby/Elsevier, Edinburgh

Eble JN, Sauter G, Epstein JE, Sesterhenn IA (eds) (2004) World Health Organization classification of tumors: pathology and genetics. Tumours of the urinary system and male genital organs. IARC Press, Lyon

Murphy WM, Grignon DJ, Perlman EJ (2004) Tumors of the kidney, bladder, and related urinary structures. 4th series. Armed Forces Institute of Pathology, Washington, DC

Articles

1. Delahunt B (2009) Advances and controversies in grading and staging of renal cell carcinoma. Mod Pathol 22:s24–s36
2. Srigely JR, Hutter RVP, Gelb AB (1997) Current prognostic factors-renal cell carcinoma. Cancer 80:994–996
3. Fuhrman SA, Lasky LC, Lima C (1982) Prognostic significance of morphologic parameters in renal cell carcinoma. Am J Surg Pathol 6:655–663
4. Serano MF, Katz M, Yan Y et al (2008) Percentage of high-grade carcinoma as a prognostic indicator in patients with renal cell carcinoma. Cancer 113:477–483
5. Nese N, Paner G, Mallin K et al (2009) Renal cell carcinoma: assessment of key pathologic prognostic parameters and patient characteristics in 47 909 cases using National Cancer Data Base. Ann Diagn Pathol 13:1–8
6. Brookman-May S, May M, Zigeuner R et al (2011) Collecting system invasion and Fuhrman grade but not tumor size facilitate prognostic stratification of patients with pT2 renal cell carcinoma. J Urol 186:2175–2181
7. Al-Aynati M, Chen V, Salama S et al (2003) Interobserver and intraobserver variability using the Fuhrman grading system for renal cell carcinoma. Arch Pathol Lab Med 127:593–596
8. Sun M, Lunghezzani G, Jeldres C et al (2009) A proposal for reclassification of the Fuhrman grading system in patients with clear cell renal cell carcinoma. Eur Urol 56:775–781
9. Delahunt B, Sika-Paotonu D, Bethwaite PB et al (2011) Grading of clear cell renal cell carcinoma should be based on nucleolar prominence. Am J Surg Pathol 35:1134–1139
10. Higgins JP, McKenney JK, Brooks JD et al (2009) Recommendations for the reporting of surgically resected specimens of renal cell carcinoma. The Association of Directors of Anatomic and Surgical Pathology. Hum Pathol 40:456–463
11. Chapman-Fredricks JR, Herrera L, Bracho J et al (2011) Adult renal cell carcinoma with rhabdoid morphology represents a neoplastic dedifferentiation analogous to sarcomatoid carcinoma. Ann Diagn Pathol 15:333–337
12. Algaba F, Akaza H, Lopez-Beltran A et al (2011) Current pathology keys of renal cell carcinoma. Eur Urol 60:634–643
13. Sukov WR, Lohse CM, Leibovich BC et al (2012) Clinical and pathological features associated with prognosis in patients with papillary renal cell carcinoma. J Urol 187:54–59
14. Delahunt B, Eble JN (1997) Papillary renal cell carcinoma: a clinicopathologic and immunohistochemical study of 105 tumors. Mod Pathol 10:537–544
15. Steffens S, Janssen M, Roos FC et al (2012) Incidence and long-term prognosis of papillary compared to renal cell carcinoma- a multicentre study. Eur J Cancer 48:2347–2352
16. Klatte T, Anterasian C, Said JW et al (2010) Fuhrman grade provides higher prognostic accuracy than nucleolar grade for papillary renal cell carcinoma. J Urol 183:2143–2147
17. Sika-Paotonu D, Bethwaite PB, McCredie MR et al (2006) Nucleolar grade but not Fuhrman grade is applicable to papillary renal cell carcinoma. Am J Surg Pathol 30:1091–1096
18. Amin M, Paner GP, Alvarado-Cabrero I et al (2008) Chromophobe renal cell carcinoma: histomorphologic characteristics and evaluation of conventional prognostic parameters in 145 cases. Am J Surg Pathol 32:1822–1834
19. Finley DS, Shuch B, Said JW et al (2011) The chromophobe tumor grading system is the preferred grading scheme for chromophobe renal cell carcinoma. J Urol 186:2168–2174
20. Delahunt B, Sika-Paotonu D, Bethwaite PB et al (2007) Fuhrman grading is not appropriate for chromophobe renal cell carcinoma. Am J Surg Pathol 31:957–960
21. Paner G, Amin MB, Alvarado-Cabrero I et al (2010) A novel tumor grading scheme for chromophobe renal cell carcinoma prognostic utility and comparison with Fuhrman nuclear grade. Am J Surg Pathol 34:1233–1240
22. Przybycin CG, Cronin AM, Darvishian F et al (2011) Chromophobe renal cell carcinoma: a clinicopathologic study of 203 tumors in 200 patients with primary resection at a single institution. Am J Surg Pathol 35:962–970
23. Cheville JC, Lohse CM, Sukov WR et al (2012) Chromophobe renal cell carcinoma: the impact of tumor grade on outcome. Am J Surg Pathol 36:851–856

24. Gupta R, Billis A, Shah RB et al (2012) Carcinoma of the collecting ducts of Bellini and renal medullary carcinoma: clinicopathologic analysis of 52 cases of rare aggressive subtypes of renal cell carcinoma with a focus on their interrelationship. Am J Surg Pathol 36:1265–1278

25. Lopez-Beltran A, Kirkali Z, Montironi R et al (2012) Unclassified renal cell carcinoma: a report of 56 cases. BJU Int 110:786–793

26. Perez-Montiel D, Wakerly PE Jr, Hes O et al (2006) High grade urothelial carcinoma of the renal pelvis: clinicopathologic study of 108 cases with emphasis on unusual morphologic variants. Mod Pathol 19:494–503

27. Young A, Kunju LP (2012) High grade carcinomas involving the renal sinus. Report of a case and review of the differential diagnosis and immunohistochemical expression. Arch Pathol Lab Med 136:907–910

28. Klatte T, Streubel B, Wrba F et al (2012) Renal cell carcinoma associated with transcription factor E3 expression and Xp11.2 translocation. Incidence, characteristics and prognosis. Am J Clin Pathol 137:761–768

29. Amin MB, Gupta R, Hes O et al (2009) Primary thyroid-like follicular carcinoma of the kidney: report of 6 cases of a histologically distinctive adult renal epithelial neoplasm. Am J Surg Pathol 33:393–400

30. Alessandrini L, Fassan M, Gardiman MP et al (2012) Thyroid-like follicular carcinoma of the kidney: report of two cases with detailed immunohistochemical profile and literature review. Virchows Arch 461: 345–350

31. Fine SW, Argani P, DeMarzo AM et al (2006) Expanding the histologic spectrum of mucinous tubular and spindle cell carcinoma of the kidney. Am J Surg Pathol 30:1554–1560

32. Shen SS, Ro JY, Tamboli P et al (2007) Mucinous tubular and spindle cell carcinoma of kidney is probably a variant of papillary renal cell carcinoma with spindle cell features. Ann Diagn Pathol 11: 13–21

33. Ursani NA, Robertson AR, Schieman SM (2011) Mucinous tubular and spindle cell carcinoma of kidney without sarcomatoid change showing metastases to liver and retroperitoneal lymph node. Hum Pathol 42:444–448

Tumors of the Urinary Bladder

8

Liang Cheng, Gregory T. MacLennan,
and Antonio Lopez-Beltran

8.1   Introduction

Nearly half of all bladder tumors are noninvasive (stage pTa) papillary neoplasms of urothelial origin. These tumors have been intensively investigated for many decades, and a number of concepts regarding their biologic behavior and prognosis have been well established. Prognosis for these tumors is influenced by tumor size, tumor multifocality, recurrence status, coexistence of carcinoma in situ, and histologic tumor grade [1–6]. The first four elements are straightforward. However, there has been a long-standing lack of agreement among pathologists concerning the ideal system for grading these tumors. A uniform grading system for bladder cancer will allow for valid comparison of treatment results among different centers. The 1973 WHO classification is preferred by some authors because it allows comparison of results between different clinical centers. It is a robust, time-tested, and reasonably reproducible method for pathologic reporting of bladder tumors. The 1998 WHO/ISUP classification of bladder tumors, and its adoption in

L. Cheng, M.D. (✉)
Department of Pathology and Laboratory Medicine,
Indiana University School of Medicine,
Indianapolis, IN, USA
e-mail: liang_cheng@yahoo.com

G.T. MacLennan, M.D.
Institute of Pathology, Case Western Reserve University,
Cleveland, OH, USA

A. Lopez-Beltran, M.D., Ph.D.
Department of Surgery, Unit of Anatomic Pathology,
Cordoba University School of Medicine, Cordoba, Spain

the 2004 WHO classification, has been the subject of considerable controversy [3, 7–28]. In particular, there is poor interobserver agreement in the diagnostic categories of papillary urothelial neoplasm of low malignant potential (PUNLMP) and low-grade urothelial carcinoma, two new categories in the 2004 WHO system [8, 9, 12, 29–34]. Use of both the 1973 and 2004 WHO classifications (former 1998 ISUP/WHO) has been recommended by some [3, 8, 11, 12, 35–37]. We recently introduced a new four-tiered grading system, which expands previous grading systems to include an additional category of noninvasive papillary carcinomas with exceptionally abnormal cytologic characteristics (Fig. 8.1, Table 8.1) [38]. This new grading system has the combined strengths of both 1973 WHO and 2004 WHO grading system [38].

8.2   Historical Perspective

In the 1973 WHO classification of urothelial tumors, papillary urothelial neoplasms were separated into four categories: papilloma and carcinoma grades 1–3 [39]. Papillomas were defined as exophytic tumors consisting of delicate fibrovascular cores covered by normal looking urothelium with intact umbrella cells and virtually lacking mitotic activity. Clinically, these tumors are typically solitary and less than 1.0 cm in diameter, occur in patients less than 50 years old, and have a negligible recurrence rate [40]. Regarding tumors diagnosed as carcinoma, histologic grading was based on the degree of cellular anaplasia, with

I. Damjanov, F. Fan (eds.), *Cancer Grading Manual*,
DOI 10.1007/978-3-642-34516-6_8, © Springer-Verlag Berlin Heidelberg 2013

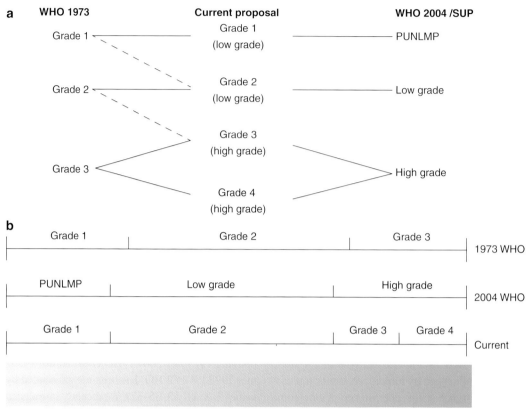

Histologic spectrum of urothelial carcinoma

Fig. 8.1 Comparisons of different grading systems. (**a**) The 1973 WHO grade 1 carcinomas are reassigned, some to the papillary urothelial neoplasm of low malignant potential (*PUNLMP*) category and some to the low-grade carcinoma category in the 2004 WHO classification. Similarly, 1973 WHO grade 2 carcinomas are reassigned, some to the low-grade carcinoma category and others to the high-grade carcinoma category. All 1973 WHO grade 3 tumors are assigned to the high-grade carcinoma category. In the current proposal, PUNLMP has been reassigned as grade 1 carcinoma, 2004 low-grade urothelial carcinoma has been reassigned as grade 2 urothelial carcinoma, and 2004 high-grade urothelial carcinoma has been divided into grade 3 and grade 4 urothelial carcinomas (*all high grade*). Grade 4 urothelial carcinomas are more commonly associated with invasion. (**b**) Urothelial carcinomas encompass a continuous spectrum of diseases with various biologic behavior and morphologic manifestations. Defining exact cutoff for each disease category can be challenging. *WHO* World Health Organization, *ISUP* International Society of Urological Pathology, *PUNLMP* papillary urothelial neoplasm of low malignant potential (From Ref. [38], with permission)

Table 8.1 Grading of urothelial carcinoma of the urinary bladder

1973 WHO	1998 WHO/ISUP	1999 WHO	2004 WHO	Current proposal
Papilloma	Papilloma	Papilloma	Papilloma	Papilloma
Grade 1	PUNLMP	PUNLMP	PUNLMP	Grade 1 (low grade)
Grade 2	Low grade	Grade 1	Low grade	Grade 2 (low grade)
		Grade 2		Grade 3 (high grade)
Grade 3	High grade	Grade 3	High grade	Grade 4 (high grade)

Note: All the grading schemes have substantial inter- and intraobserver variabilities. There is no exact correlation between different grading systems. Some 1973 WHO grade 2 tumors are "low grade," and some are classified as "high grade." The 1998 WHO/ISUP system is the same as the 2004 WHO system

Abbreviations: *WHO* World Health Organization, *IUSP* International Society of Urological Pathology, *PUNLMP* papillary urothelial neoplasm of low malignant potential grade 1 tumors having the least degree of anaplasia compatible with a diagnosis of malignancy, grade 3 tumors having the most severe degree of anaplasia, and grade 2 tumors having an intermediate degree of cellular anaplasia [39]. Anaplasia was further defined in the 1973 WHO classification as increased cellularity, nuclear crowding, disturbances of cellular polarity, failure of differentiation from the base to the surface, polymorphism, irregularity in the size of cells, variations of shape and chromatin pattern of the nuclei, displaced or abnormal mitotic figures, and giant cells [39].

A recurring criticism of the 1973 WHO grading system is that it did not define distinct cutoff points between the three tumor grades. At opposite ends of the spectrum of anaplasia, a pathologist may have little difficulty assigning a tumor as either grade 1 or grade 3 carcinoma. Distinguishing grade 2 carcinoma from grade 1 carcinoma at one end of the spectrum and from grade 3 carcinoma at the opposite end of the spectrum is the most difficult aspect of applying the 1973 WHO grading system, with the result that there is wide variation in the reported frequency of grade 2 carcinoma and with reported incidences ranging from 13–69 % [10]. This has raised concerns about lack of reproducibility in assigning tumor grades, and with this came concerns about the appropriateness of certain clinical management stratagems in a setting of uncertainty about proper tumor grade. Despite its apparent shortcomings, the 1973 WHO grading system has been in widespread use for more than three decades. It is accepted by uropathologists and uro-oncologists on a global scale. Enormous amounts of data have been accumulated using this system in studies of the morphologic properties, clinical behavior, treatment, and follow-up of urothelial tumors. The system has become well understood by clinicians, who are able to tailor patient management according to the reported grades. In the opinion of many, therefore, this grading system has never been "broken," and consequently there is no apparent need to "fix it" [9].

Nevertheless, there existed a perceived need to develop a more universally acceptable classification system for bladder neoplasia that could be used effectively by pathologists, urologists, and oncologists. Consequently, following an initial meeting in 1997 between pathologists, urologists, and basic scientists in Washington, D.C., at which it was agreed that an attempt would be made to create such a system, several members of the International Society of Urologic Pathologists (ISUP) in 1998 proposed a new grading system, subsequently known as the 1998 WHO/ISUP system. A revised version of this system (the 1999 WHO/ISUP system) met with limited acceptance. At a consensus conference in 2001, the majority opinion of the participants was that the 1973 WHO grading system should remain the international standard for the classification and grading of urothelial papillary neoplasms [10]. In 2004, a classification system for noninvasive papillary urothelial neoplasms, identical to the 1998 WHO/ISUP classification system, was adopted in *Pathology and Genetics of Tumours of the Urinary System and Male Genital Organs*, one of a series of WHO "Blue Books" for the classification of tumors. This new system separates noninvasive papillary urothelial neoplasms into four categories, designated papilloma, papillary urothelial neoplasm of low malignant potential (PUNLMP), low-grade carcinoma, and high-grade carcinoma.

The authors of the new 2004 WHO classification system expressed hope and expectation that the new system would be widely accepted among all physicians affected by the system. A striking feature of the new system was the introduction of a newly designated category, PUNLMP, in order to circumvent use of the term carcinoma for tumors with a low probability of progression, but yet not entirely benign. It was emphasized in the introduction of this new system that it provides detailed histologic criteria for the diagnosis of papillary urothelial neoplasms, a feature that was expected to improve diagnostic reproducibility among pathologists. Additionally, it was anticipated that there would be reasonable consistency with the terminology used in urinary cytology, allowing easier cytohistologic correlation and improved patient management.

8.3 Histologic Grading According to the 1973 WHO Classification

Histologic grading is one of the most important prognostic factors in bladder cancer. The first widely accepted grading system for papillary urothelial neoplasms was the WHO (1973) classification system, as already stated. The histologic criteria for the diagnostic categories in the 1973 WHO classification are described in the following sections.

8.3.1 Urothelial Papilloma

Urothelial papilloma is a benign exophytic neoplasm composed of a delicate fibrovascular core covered by normal appearing urothelium [40]. The superficial cells are often prominent. Mitoses are absent or, if present, located in the basal cell layer. The stroma may show edema and inflammatory cells [40]. Papillomas are diploid with low proliferation, uncommon p53 expression, and frequent FGFR3 (75 %) mutation. Cytokeratin (CK) 20 expression is limited to the superficial (umbrella) cells as in normal urothelium. Papilloma accounts for less than 1 % of all bladder tumors and the male to female ratio is 1.9:1. Hematuria is common. Most papillomas are single and occur in younger patients (mean age, 46 years), close to the ureteric orifices. Urothelial papillomas may recur but do not progress.

8.3.2 1973 WHO Grade 1 Urothelial Carcinoma

Grade 1 papillary urothelial carcinoma consists of an orderly arrangement of normal urothelial cells lining delicate papillae with minimal architectural abnormality and minimal nuclear atypia. Grade 1 urothelial carcinoma appears to have a predilection for the ureteric orifices. In one study, 69 % of grade 1 urothelial carcinomas were centered near a ureteric orifice, but the remainder was seen in all other portions of the bladder. Patients with grade 1 urothelial carcinoma are at increased risk of local recurrence, progression, and dying of bladder cancer. Significant morbidity and mortality are associated with grade 1 urothelial carcinoma of the bladder if patients are followed up for a sufficient interval [41–54]. With 20 years of follow-up, Holmang et al. [43] found that 14 % of patients with noninvasive grade 1 urothelial carcinoma (pTa G1) died of bladder cancer. In a recent review

of 152 patients with stage Ta grade 1 urothelial carcinoma, Leblanc et al. found that 83 patients (55 %) had tumor recurrence, including 37 % with cancer progression [45]. Patients who remained tumor-free for 1 year still had a 43 % chance of late recurrence. In Greene's study of 100 patients with grade 1 urothelial carcinoma, ten patients (10 %) died of bladder cancer after more than 15 years; of 73 patients who had recurrences, 22 % were of higher grade than the original tumor [55]. The mean interval from diagnosis to development of invasive cancer was 8 years. Jordan et al. studied 91 patients with grade 1 papillary urothelial tumors and found that 40 % had recurrence. Twenty percent of patients with recurrences developed high-grade (grade 3) cancer, and four patients (4 %) died of bladder cancer [53]. Long-term follow-up is recommended for patients with grade 1 papillary urothelial carcinoma.

8.3.3 1973 WHO Grade 2 Urothelial Carcinoma

Grade 2 urothelial carcinoma represents a broad group of tumors encompassing a spectrum of cytologic atypia and some variability in the relative proportion of cells with atypical features. Grade 2 urothelial carcinomas retain some of the overall maturation of grade 1 carcinoma but also display at least focal moderate variation in polarity, nuclear appearance, and chromatin texture apparent at low magnification. The prognosis for patients with grade 2 urothelial carcinoma is significantly worse than for those with lower-grade papillary cancer [10, 13, 56]. Recurrence risk for patients with noninvasive grade 2 urothelial carcinoma is 45–67 % [10, 13, 56]. Invasion occurs in up to 20 %, and cancer-specific death is expected in 13–20 % following surgical treatment. Patients with grade 2 urothelial carcinoma and lamina propria invasion are at even greater risk, with recurrences in 67–80 % of cases, the development of muscle invasive cancer in 21–49 %, and cancer-specific death in 17–51 % of those treated surgically [10, 13, 56]. Some authors consider both nuclear pleomorphism and mitotic count as criteria for subdividing grade 2 urothelial carcinoma (grades 2A and 2B), and they have been successful in identifying groups of cancers with different outcomes [25, 57–60]. However, subclassification of grade 2 urothelial carcinoma is not recommended due to significant interobserver variability.

8.3.4   1973 WHO Grade 3 Urothelial Carcinoma

Grade 3 urothelial carcinoma displays the most extreme nuclear abnormality of any papillary urothelial cancer, similar to changes observed in urothelial carcinoma in situ. Cellular anaplasia, characteristic of grade 3 urothelial carcinoma, is defined as increased cellularity, nuclear crowding, random cellular polarity, absence of normal mucosal differentiation, nuclear pleomorphism, irregularity in cell size, variation in nuclear shape, capricious chromatin pattern, increased frequency of mitotic figures, and occasional neoplastic giant cells [39]. Recurrence risk for patients with noninvasive grade 3 urothelial carcinoma is 65–85 %, with invasion occurring in 20–52 %, and cancer-specific death in up to 35 % following surgical treatment [56, 61]. Of surgically treated patients with grade 3 urothelial carcinoma and lamina propria invasion, 46–71 % develop recurrences, 24–48 % develop muscle invasive cancer, and 25–71 % suffer cancer-specific death, emphasizing a need for aggressive treatment of these patients [10, 11, 13].

8.4   Histologic Grading According to the 1998 ISUP/2004 WHO Classification

8.4.1   Urothelial Papilloma

The diagnostic criteria and terminology are identical to those of the 1973 WHO classification [39, 62].

8.4.2   Papillary Urothelial Neoplasm of Low Malignant Potential

PUNLMP is a low-grade urothelial tumor with a papillary architecture and a purported low incidence

of recurrence and progression [7–9, 11, 63–65]. This lesion is histologically defined by the WHO 2004 classification system as a papillary urothelial tumor that resembles the exophytic urothelial papilloma, but with increased cellular proliferation exceeding the thickness of normal urothelium. All such tumors would be grade 1 urothelial carcinomas by the WHO 1973 grading system. Clinically, these tumors show a male predominance (3:1) and occur at a mean age of 65 years [66]. They are most commonly identified during investigation of gross or microscopic hematuria. Cystoscopically, these lesions are typically 1–2 cm in greatest dimension and located on the lateral wall of the bladder or near the ureteric orifices [66]. They have been described as having a "seaweed in the ocean" appearance.

PUNLMP has high recurrence but low progression incidence. Recurrence and progression rates were 18 % and 2 %, respectively, for PUNLMP in a recent study [67]. In another study, Samaratunga et al. found that PUNLMP and low-grade urothelial carcinoma had progression rates of 8 % and 13 %, respectively [68]. Similar recurrence and stage progression results were subsequently found in additional studies. The tumor recurrence rate after the diagnosis of PUNLMP was reported to be 35 % in the study by Holmang et al. [69] and 47 % in the study by Pich et al. [16]. Holmang et al. concluded that PUNLMP and low-grade carcinoma have similar risks of progression when compared to high-grade carcinoma [69]. In a study of 53 PUNLMP tumors with a mean follow-up period of 11.7 years, Fujii et al. reported a recurrence rate of 60 %, with 34 % progressing to low-grade carcinoma and 8 % progressing to invasive carcinoma (stage T1) [20]. In a study of 322 patients with a mean follow-up period of 6.6 years, Oosterhuis et al. [17] found no difference with regard to tumor recurrence or disease progression between patients with PUNLMP and patients with low-grade urothelial carcinoma. They concluded that there are insufficient data to justify a different clinical approach or the introduction of a new pathologic category. Samaratunga et al. [68] studied 134 patients with noninvasive papillary urothelial tumors from Johns Hopkins Hospital and found that both the WHO 1973 and WHO (2004)/ISUP grading systems were predictive of patient outcome

($P=0.003$ and $P=0.002$, respectively). However, their reported progression rate to invasive disease for patients with PUNLMP was the highest of any published study [8, 9]. With a median follow-up of 56 months, the 1973 WHO grade 1 tumors were found to have a progression rate of 11 %, whereas the WHO (2004)/ISUP PUNLMP tumors were found to have a progression rate of 8 % [68]. Lee et al. found 42 % of PUNLMP had tumor recurrence and 29 % progressed to higher tumor grade [70]. These data indicate that patients with PUNLMP do not have a benign neoplasm but instead have significant risk of tumor recurrence and disease progression. Clinical studies to determine an optimal length and frequency of follow-up in these patients would be especially important, given that the reported mean interval from initial diagnosis of PUNLMP to development of invasive carcinoma was 13 years [66]. Long-term clinical follow-up is recommended for these patients.

The greatest source of controversy with the WHO (2004)/ISUP classification system centers on the diagnosis of PUNLMP [5, 10, 13, 17, 30, 71]. Some authors consider PUNLMP to be an essentially benign tumor with a negligible progression rate. However, others feel that PUNLMP terminology increases the complexity of histologic grading and does not accurately reflect biological potential. Since PUNLMP is a low-grade papillary urothelial tumor with a substantial incidence of recurrence and reported progression rates that are relatively low but nonetheless very comparable to those of low-grade urothelial carcinoma, some investigators have questioned the rationale of separating these tumors from neoplasms diagnosed previously as grade 1 urothelial carcinomas using the criteria of the WHO 1973 grading system.

8.4.3   2004 WHO Low-Grade Urothelial Carcinoma

A low-grade papillary urothelial carcinoma shows fronds with recognizable variation in architecture and cytology [11, 62]. The tumor consists of slender papillae with frequent branching and variation in nuclear polarity. The nuclei show enlargement and irregularity with vesicular

chromatin, and nucleoli are often present. Mitotic figures may occur at any level in low-grade papillary urothelial carcinoma. Such cases would have been considered as grade 1 or grade 2 carcinomas in the WHO 1973 classification scheme. Altered expression of CK20, CD44, p53, and p63 is frequent. Some tumors are diploid, but aneuploidy is the rule. FGFR3 mutations are seen with about the same frequency as in PUNLMP [11, 12, 14, 62]. The male to female ratio is 2.9:1, and the mean age is 70 years (range, 28–90 years). Most patients present with hematuria and have a single tumor in the posterior or lateral bladder wall. However, 22 % of patients with low-grade papillary urothelial carcinoma have two or more tumors. Tumor recurrence, stage progression, and tumor-related mortality are 50 %, 10 %, and 4 %, respectively. In another series of 215 patients with low-grade noninvasive papillary urothelial carcinoma, 17 patients (8 %) had grade or stage progression and one patient (0.5 %) died of bladder cancer [72]. Grade and stage progression occurred in 18 % and 7 % of patients, respectively, in another study [73]. Pellucchi and colleagues were able to further stratify 2004 WHO low-grade urothelial carcinomas into two separate risk groups using the 1973 WHO grading scheme [74]. According to the 1973 WHO grading system, 87 low-grade (2004 WHO) tumors (32 %) were classified as 1973 WHO grade 1 tumors, and 183 low-grade (2004 WHO) tumors (68 %) were classified as 1973 WHO grade 2 tumors among 270 consecutive patients with a first episode of low-grade pTa bladder cancer at transurethral resection of the bladder between 2004 and 2008. Five-year recurrence-free survival rate was 49 % for the low-grade population and 62 % and 40 % for the 1973 WHO grade 1 and grade 2 groups, respectively [74].

8.4.4   2004 WHO High-Grade Urothelial Carcinoma

In high-grade papillary urothelial carcinoma, the cells lining the papillary fronds show obviously disordered arrangement with cytologic atypia. All tumors classified as grade 3 in the 1973 WHO schema, as well as some tumors assigned grade 2 in that classification, would be considered high-grade carcinoma in the 2004 WHO classification. The papillae are frequently fused. Both architectural and cytologic abnormalities are recognizable at scanning power [11]. The nuclei are pleomorphic with prominent nucleoli and altered polarity. Mitotic figures are frequent. The thickness of the urothelium varies considerably. Carcinoma in situ is frequently evident in the adjacent mucosa. Changes in CK20, p53, and p63 expression, as well as aneuploidy, are more frequent than in low-grade neoplasms. Molecular alterations in these tumors include overexpression of p53, HER2, or EGFR, and loss of p21Waf1 or p27kip1 as seen with invasive cancers. Genetically, high-grade noninvasive neoplasms (pTa G3) resemble invasive carcinomas [11, 62]. A comparative genomic hybridization study showed deletions at 2q, 5q, 10q, and 18q as well as gains at 5p and 20q [75]. Hematuria is common and the endoscopic appearance varies from papillary to nodular or solid. There may be single or multiple tumors. Stage progression and death due to disease are observed in as many as 65 % of patients [8, 11, 62]. In a recent analysis of 85 patients with Ta high-grade urothelial carcinoma, recurrence and tumor progression rates were 37 % and 40 %, respectively [76].

8.4.4.1 Comments

Interobserver Variability and Reproducibility

All grading systems are hampered by varying degrees of subjectivity that affect interobserver reproducibility. Published reports of the reproducibility of grading systems are often derived from the efforts of small groups of pathologists, who have previously worked or trained together; consequently, interobserver variation between pathologists unfamiliar with one another may be even greater than between such small groups. An important goal of the 2004 WHO classification was to provide detailed explanations of the histologic criteria for each diagnostic category and thereby improve reproducibility between different pathologists.

Despite provision of detailed histologic criteria for the diagnostic categories in the 2004 WHO system, improvement in intraobserver and

interobserver variability as compared to the 1973 WHO system has not been documented [30–34]. In fact, Mikuz demonstrated that interobserver agreement was higher using the 1973 WHO classification than when using either the 2004 WHO or 1999 WHO/ISUP systems [23]. In a study by Yorokoglu and colleagues [27], the intraobserver and interobserver reproducibility of both the 2004 WHO and the 1973 WHO systems were evaluated by assigning six urologic pathologists to the task of independently reviewing 30 slides of noninvasive papillary urothelial tumors in a study set. They found no statistical difference between the reproducibility achieved with either system; the new system failed to improve reproducibility [27]. There was agreement for PUNLMP in only 48 % of cases and reproducibility was lower for low-grade tumors in both the 2004 WHO and the 1973 WHO systems [27]. Murphy et al. recorded a 50 % discrepancy rate among pathologists attempting to distinguish between PUNLMP and low-grade papillary urothelial carcinoma after a period of structured pathologist education [29]. In several studies, several pathologists have refused to make a diagnosis of PUNLMP [32, 34].

In fairness, reproducibility in the 1973 WHO classification of urothelial tumors is also problematic. A frequent criticism of this classification scheme is that the morphologic criteria proposed for grading these neoplasms are vague and ill defined, particularly those used in separating the three grades of carcinoma. No distinct cutoff points between the three tumor grades were defined in the 1973 WHO classification system, resulting in lack of agreement among pathologists concerning the proper assignment of grade in noninvasive urothelial tumors. At opposite ends of the spectrum of anaplasia, a pathologist may have little difficulty assigning a tumor as either grade 1 or grade 3 carcinoma. Distinguishing grade 2 carcinoma from grade 1 carcinoma at one end of the spectrum and from grade 3 carcinoma at the opposite end is the most difficult aspect of applying the 1973 WHO grading system, resulting in a wide variation in the reported frequency of grade 2 carcinoma, with reported incidences ranging from 13–69 %. This is often mentioned as a major shortcoming of the WHO 1973 grading system, one that justifies the creation of a new improved grading system [10]. It is ironic, however, in several separate publications in which noninvasive papillary urothelial tumors were graded according to the WHO/ISUP system, the incidence of PUNLMP varied from 6–62 %, that of low-grade carcinoma varied from 27–77 %, and the incidence of high-grade carcinoma varied from 15–74 % [16, 17, 28, 63, 67–69, 72, 77–84]. In a recent analysis of 270 consecutive patients with a diagnosis of low-grade noninvasive papillary urothelial carcinoma between 2004 and 2008, only 20 patients were diagnosed with PUNLMP during the same study period [74]. Both the 1973 and the 2004 WHO grading systems are hampered by the fact that there is considerable heterogeneity within papillary urothelial neoplasms, making the assignment of a single grade to a tumor problematic in many instances [25, 85]. Regardless of the terminology or classification systems used, noninvasive papillary urothelial carcinoma should be considered as a disease with a wide spectrum of biological and morphological manifestations. Given the high interobserver variability and significant overlap between PUNLMP and low-grade urothelial carcinoma, it may not be justifiable to create a separate disease category ("PUNLMP") with an appellation that implies that the entity described has striking biological difference from low-grade noninvasive papillary urothelial carcinoma and therefore can be managed differently than might be expected if an unequivocal diagnosis of carcinoma (low-grade noninvasive papillary urothelial carcinoma) were rendered.

8.5 Histologic Grading of Urothelial Carcinoma: Current Proposal

The histopathologic grade of urothelial tumors is one of the best predictors of biological behavior. The criteria for pathologic grading of noninvasive papillary urothelial neoplasms have been a source of controversy for many decades [86]. Numerous classification schemes have been proposed, but the most widely accepted and used is the 1973 WHO classification [39]. The major criticism of this classification scheme is vague and poorly defined morphologic criteria for grading these neoplasms. Because no clearly defined cutoff points between the different grades were defined in the WHO 1973 classification system, there is considerable debate among pathologists concerning the proper assignment of grade in noninvasive urothelial tumors, especially those falling into the grade 1 and grade 2 categories. This has resulted in a lumping of cases into the grade 2 category with a wide range of reported incidences for grade 2 carcinomas, ranging from 13–69 % [10]. There is inevitably a degree of heterogeneity within the grades when comparing studies using the WHO 1973 classification.

In 1998, the WHO and the ISUP proposed a new consensus classification system intended to provide better morphologic criteria for grading, to achieve better standardization, and to avoid using the term "carcinoma" for tumors with a very low probability of progressing or recurring [87]. The diagnostic category of PUNLMP was created to achieve these goals. In 1999, within a 12-month period from publication of the WHO/ISUP 1998 system, the WHO again changed their preferred classification system (WHO 1999) to closely mirror the three-tiered WHO 1973 grading system preserving PUNLMP as the lowest risk category [88]. Considering the above discussion on the biologic behavior and the molecular characteristics of PUNLMP, it seems evident that PUNLMP is an indolent variety of what we generally regard as "carcinoma." A diagnosis of PUNLMP implies a real and significant potential for an adverse clinical outcome that does not differ greatly from that of 2004 WHO low-grade noninvasive urothelial carcinomas. In a series of 504 patients with noninvasive urothelial tumors, several studies found no clear advantage of the 2004 WHO grading system over the 1973 WHO grading system [28, 89]. With a mean follow-up of 7.2 years (range, 3–11 years), 5-year survival for PUNLMP (94 %) was essentially identical to that of low-grade urothelial carcinoma (93 %) [28].

A great deal of the confusion and controversy regarding the proper histologic grading of bladder tumors stems from the fact that the term "carcinoma" is routinely used to describe noninvasive neoplasms in this organ. Nonetheless, the term "carcinoma" or "adenocarcinoma" has also been used to describe tumors without evidence of invasion in other organ systems (e.g., uterus) as well. Another criticism of the WHO 1973 classification of urothelial tumors is that very low-grade noninvasive tumors with a low probability of progressing are labeled as "carcinomas," consequently, subjecting patients with these tumors to psychosocial stigma as well as financial and insurance consequences that follow a diagnosis of cancer. Indeed, the creation of the diagnostic category of PUNLMP was designed, in part, to free patients with this diagnosis from these burdens. However, as detailed above, PUNLMP has a reported recurrence rate up to 60 % and a progression rate up to 8 % [17–20, 68]. Thus, a diagnosis of PUNLMP carries with it a real and significant potential for an adverse clinical outcome similar to that of low-grade noninvasive urothelial carcinomas, as defined by the WHO (2004)/ISUP classification system. Claims that PUNLMP is benign should be viewed within the context of length of follow-up. Speculations about the psychosocial burdens of a carcinoma diagnosis are unproven. On the other hand, some noninvasive papillary urothelial carcinomas (both low grade and high grade) may never recur or progress after removal. Why then do these tumors warrant a designation as "carcinoma" in the WHO (2004)/ISUP classification when many behave as an indolent tumor? A greater understanding of urothelial tumor genetics and of clinical diagnostic applications may eventually discern which genetic derangements are responsible for aggressive biological behavior [6]. This molecular prognostic detail would allow pathologists to sort out which noninvasive tumors should be called "carcinoma." However, until that time, it seems prudent to treat PUNLMP as a low-grade noninvasive carcinoma and follow these patients closely. In the study by Samaratunga et al., a statistically significant difference in progression rates was seen for PUNLMP (8 %) and low-grade noninvasive urothelial carcinoma (13 %). However, based on high reported rates of interobserver variability when diagnosing PUNLMP, it may not be necessary

or clinically justified to create a distinct diagnostic category for these low-grade urothelial tumors. Accumulated data suggest that PUNLMP should be treated in a manner similar to low-grade noninvasive carcinoma. In the current proposal, noninvasive papillary urothelial tumors are separated into five categories: papilloma, grade 1 urothelial carcinoma (low grade), grade 2 urothelial carcinoma (low grade), grade 3 urothelial carcinoma (high grade), and grade 4 urothelial carcinoma (high grade) (Tables 8.1, 8.2, and 8.3; Fig. 8.1). PUNLMP is classified as "grade 1 urothelial carcinoma (low grade)" [38].

8.5.1 Urothelial Papilloma

The diagnostic criteria and terminology are identical to those defined in the 1973 and 2004 WHO classification [39, 62].

8.5.2 Grade 1 Urothelial Carcinoma (Low Grade)

The diagnostic criteria are identical to those defined in the 1998 WHO/ISUP and 2004 WHO classification for PUNLMP. We propose to change the terminology of PUNLMP to "grade 1 urothelial carcinoma (low grade)." In these tumors, cytologic atypia is minimal or absent and architectural abnormalities are slight with preserved polarity. Mitotic figures are infrequent and usually limited to the basal layer. Grade 1 tumor should be distinguished from urothelial papilloma, which is a benign lesion without invasive potential or risk of progression. The key difference between papilloma and grade 1 urothelial carcinoma (low grade) is the number of epithelial layers covering the papillae (Fig. 8.2a, Tables 8.2 and 8.3) [66].

8.5.3 Grade 2 Urothelial Carcinoma (Low Grade)

The diagnostic criteria are identical to those defined in the 1998 WHO/ISUP and 2004 WHO classification for low-grade urothelial carcinomas.

Table 8.2 Diagnostic criteria for the newly proposed grading system of urothelial carcinoma of the bladder

Characteristics	Grade 1 (low grade)	Grade 2 (low grade)	Grade 3 (high grade)	Grade 4 (high grade)
Increased cell layers (>7)	Yes	Variable	Variable	Variable, usually <7 layers
Superficial umbrella cells	Present	Often present	Usually absent	Usually absent
Polarity/overall architecture	Normal	Mildly distorted	Moderately distorted	Severely distorted
Discohesiveness	Normal	Normal	Mild to moderate	Severe
Clear cytoplasm	May be present	May be present	Usually absent	Usually absent
Nuclear size	Normal or slightly increased	Mildly increased	Moderately increased	Markedly increased
Nuclear pleomorphism	Uniform, slightly elongated to oval	Mild, round to oval with slight variation in shape and contour	Moderate	Marked
Nuclear polarization	Normal to slightly abnormal	Abnormal	Abnormal	Absent
Nuclear hyperchromasia	Slight or minimal	Mild	Moderate	Severe
Nuclear grooves	Present	Present	Absent	Absent
Nucleoli	Absent or inconspicuous	Inconspicuous	Enlarged, often prominent	Multiple prominent nucleoli
Mitotic figures	None/rare, basal location	May be present, at any level	Often present	Prominent and frequent, atypical forms
Stromal invasion	Rare	Uncommon	May be present	Often present

Note: In current proposal, grade 1 (low-grade) tumors are classified as "papillary urothelial neoplasm of low malignant potential" (*PUNLMP*) in the 2004 WHO classification system; grade 2 (low-grade) tumors are classified as "low-grade urothelial carcinoma" (2004 WHO/ISUP); grade 3 (high-grade) and grade 4 (high-grade) tumors are both classified as "high-grade urothelial carcinoma" (2004 WHO/ISUP)

Table 8.3   Differential diagnosis of urothelial papilloma and grade 1 (low-grade) urothelial carcinoma

	Urothelial papilloma	Grade 1 (low-grade) urothelial carcinoma
Age	Younger	Older
Sex (male:female)	2:1	3:1
Size	Small, usually <2 cm	Typically larger than papilloma
Microscopic findings		
Well-formed papillae	Present	Present, rarely fused
Thickness of urothelium	≤7 layers	>7 layers
Superficial umbrella cells	Present	Usually present
Cytology	Minimal or absent	Mild
Nuclear enlargement	Rare or none	None or slightly enlarged
Nuclear hyperchromasia	Rare or none	Slight or minimal
Chromatin	Fine	Fine, slightly granular
Nucleolar enlargement	Absent	Absent or inconspicuous
Nuclear pleomorphism	Absent	Absent
Mitotic figures	None	Rare or basal location
Stromal invasion	Absent	Rare

Note: Grade 1 (low-grade) urothelial carcinoma in the newly proposed grading system corresponds to those previously classified "papillary urothelial neoplasm of low malignant potential" (*PUNLMP*) in the 2004 WHO/ISUP classification system

These tumors are characterized by an overall orderly appearance but with areas of variation in architectural and cytologic features recognizable at scanning power (Table 8.2, Fig. 8.2b). They are differentiated from grade 1 urothelial carcinoma (low grade) by the presence of easily recognizable cytologic atypia including variation of polarity and nuclear size, shape, and chromatin texture. Mitotic figures are infrequent and may be seen at any level of the urothelium.

8.5.4   Grade 3 Urothelial Carcinoma (High Grade)

We feel that the spectrum of high-grade urothelial carcinomas under the 2004 WHO classification scheme is quite broad, and there is a need to separate these tumors for further investigation. Grade 3 urothelial carcinomas (high grade) display an intermediate degree of architectural and cytologic abnormality between grade 2 urothelial carcinomas (low grade) and grade 4 urothelial carcinomas (high grade) (Fig. 8.2c). Architectural disorder in these tumors is obvious, with branching and bridging of papillary projections. Nevertheless, a certain degree of polarity and nuclear uniformity are still discernible. Severe anaplasia is not seen in these tumors. All grade 3 urothelial carcinomas would be classified as high-grade urothelial carcinoma using the 2004 WHO classification scheme.

8.5.5   Grade 4 Urothelial Carcinoma (High Grade)

Cases with severe nuclear anaplasia are considered grade 4 urothelial carcinoma in the current proposal. These tumors present an overall impression of complete architectural disorder with absence of polarity, loss of superficial umbrella cells, and marked variation of all nuclear parameters (Fig. 8.2d, Table 8.2). Numerous irregularly distributed mitotic figures are frequently noted. Severe cytologic atypia is usually uniformly present in all fields or all histologic sections examined. Unlike grade 1 or grade 2 urothelial carcinoma (low grade), these tumors often have fewer than seven layers in thickness. There is remarkable cellular discohesiveness. These cases are typically associated with stromal invasion and advanced-stage bladder cancer.

Unusually aggressive variants of urothelial carcinoma, including nested variant, micropapillary variant, plasmacytoid variant, sarcomatoid carcinoma,

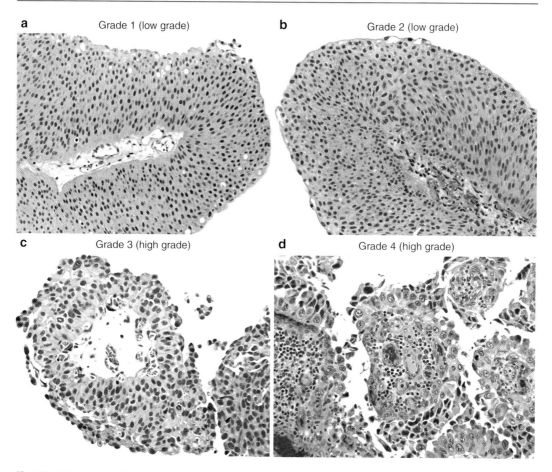

Fig. 8.2 Histologic grading of urothelial carcinoma, new proposal. (**a**) Grade 1 urothelial carcinoma (*low grade*), previously "papillary urothelial neoplasm of low malignant potential" (*PUNLMP*) (H&E stain, original magnification 200×). (**b**) Grade 2 urothelial carcinoma (*low grade*), previously low-grade urothelial carcinoma (2004 WHO classification) (H&E stain, original magnification 200×).

(**c**) Grade 3 urothelial carcinoma (*high grade*), previously high-grade urothelial carcinoma (2004 WHO classification) (H&E stain, original magnification 200×). (**d**) Grade 4 urothelial carcinoma (*high grade*), previously high-grade urothelial carcinoma (2004 WHO classification) (H&E stain, original magnification 200×) (From Ref. [38], with permission)

small-cell carcinoma, large-cell undifferentiated carcinoma, and pleomorphic giant cell carcinoma, should also be graded as grade 4 tumor in the current grading scheme.

8.5.5.1 Comment

The clinical behaviors of noninvasive papillary urothelial carcinoma are directly related to the degree of architectural, cytological, and molecular alterations of the neoplastic cells confined within the urothelium. The WHO (2004)/ISUP classification is a positive first step toward the standardization of urothelial tumor grading. Introduction of the PUNLMP category has been

the most contentious aspect of the WHO (2004)/ISUP classification of papillary bladder tumors. Studies have shown that this terminology may not reflect its true biological behavior and that interobserver variability in making this diagnosis is very high, despite detailed histologic criteria. Additionally, urine cytology in the context of the WHO (2004)/ISUP classification does not appear to effectively discriminate PUNLMP from low-grade carcinoma. For practical purposes, patients with PUNLMP should be managed according to the guidelines for management of patients with low-grade noninvasive urothelial carcinoma. Many issues have been raised regarding the use of either the 1973 WHO or the 2004 WHO grading system. We propose a four-tier grading system (grades 1–4) to replace existing grading systems. We believe that this proposed grading system incorporates the strengths of both the 1973 and the 2004 grading system. The use of both numerical (grades 1–4) and categorical schemes (low grade versus high grade) in a single grading system will allow better stratification for research purposes and facilitate clinical decision making.

References

1. Droller MJ (1998) Bladder cancer: state-of-the-art care. CA Cancer J Clin 48:269–284
2. Sylvester RJ (2006) Natural history, recurrence, and progression in superficial bladder cancer. Sci World J 6:2617–2625
3. van Rhijn BW, Burger M, Lotan Y et al (2009) Recurrence and progression of disease in non-muscle-invasive bladder cancer: from epidemiology to treatment strategy. Eur Urol 56:430–442
4. Cheng L, Neumann RM, Weaver AL et al (1999) Predicting cancer progression in patients with stage T1 bladder carcinoma. J Clin Oncol 17:3182–3187
5. Cheng L, Neumann RM, Weaver AL et al (2000) Grading and staging of bladder carcinoma in transurethral resection specimens. Correlation with 105 matched cystectomy specimens. Am J Clin Pathol 113:275–279
6. Cheng L, Zhang S, Maclennan GT et al (2011) Bladder cancer: translating molecular genetic insights into clinical practice. Hum Pathol 42:455–481
7. Montironi R, Lopez-Beltran A, Mazzucchelli R et al (2003) Classification and grading of the non-invasive urothelial neoplasms: recent advances and controversies. J Clin Pathol 56:91–95
8. MacLennan GT, Kirkali Z, Cheng L (2007) Histologic grading of noninvasive papillary urothelial neoplasms. Eur Urol 51:889–898
9. Jones TD, Cheng L (2006) Papillary urothelial neoplasm of low malignant potential: evolving terminology and concepts. J Urol 175:1995–2003
10. Bostwick DG, Mikuz G (2002) Urothelial papillary (exophytic) neoplasms. Virchows Arch 441:109–116
11. Lopez-Beltran A, Montironi R (2004) Non-invasive urothelial neoplasms: according to the most recent WHO classification. Eur Urol 46:170–176
12. Montironi R, Lopez-Beltran A, Scarpelli M et al (2009) 2004 World Health Organization classification of the noninvasive urothelial neoplasms: inherent problems and clinical reflections. Eur Urol 8:453–457
13. Bostwick DG, Ramnani D, Cheng L (1999) Diagnosis and grading of bladder cancer and associated lesions. Urol Clin North Am 26:493–507
14. Montironi R, Lopez-Beltran A, Scarpelli M et al (2008) Morphological classification and definition of benign, preneoplastic and non-invasive neoplastic lesions of the urinary bladder. Histopathology 53:621–633
15. Montironi R, Mazzucchelli R, Scarpelli M et al (2008) Morphological diagnosis of urothelial neoplasms. J Clin Pathol 61:3–10
16. Pich A, Chiusa L, Formiconi A et al (2002) Proliferative activity is the most significant predictor of recurrence in noninvasive papillary urothelial neoplasms of low malignant potential and grade 1 papillary carcinomas of the bladder. Cancer 95:784–790
17. Oosterhuis JSR, Janssen-Heijnen ML, Pauwels RP, Newling DW, ten Kate F (2002) Histological grading of papillary urothelial carcinoma of the bladder: prognostic value of the 1998 WHO/ISUP classification system and comparison with conventional grading systems. J Clin Pathol 55:900–905
18. Pich A, Chiusa L, Formiconi A et al (2001) Biologic differences between noninvasive papillary urothelial neoplasms of low malignant potential and low-grade (grade 1) papillary carcinomas of the bladder. Am J Surg Pathol 25:1528–1533
19. Holmang S, Hedelin H, Anderstrom C et al (1999) Recurrence and progression in low grade papillary urothelial tumors. J Urol 162:702–707
20. Fujii Y, Kawakami S, Koga F et al (2003) Long-term outcome of bladder papillary urothelial neoplasms of low malignant potential. BJU Int 92:559–562
21. Cheng L, MacLennan GT, Zhang S et al (2004) Laser capture microdissection analysis reveals frequent allelic losses in papillary urothelial neoplasm of low malignant potential of the urinary bladder. Cancer 101:183–188
22. Coblentz TR, Mills SE, Theodorescu D (2001) Impact of second opinion pathology in the definitive management of patients with bladder carcinoma. Cancer 91:1284–1290
23. Mikuz G (2001) The reliability and reproducibility of the different classifications of bladder cancer. In: Haupmann S, Dietel M, Sorbrinho-Simoes M (eds) Surgical pathology update 2001. ABW-Wissenschaftsverlag, Berlin, pp 114–115
24. Otto W, Denzinger S, Fritsche HM et al (2010) The WHO classification of 1973 is more suitable than the WHO classification of 2004 for predicting survival in pT1 urothelial bladder cancer. BJU Int 107:404–408
25. Cheng L, Bostwick DG (2000) World Health Organization and International Society of Urological Pathology classification and two-number grading system of bladder tumors: reply. Cancer 88:1513–1516
26. Sylvester RJ, Van der Meijden AP, Oosterlinck W et al (2006) Predicting recurrence and progression in individual patients with stage Ta T1 bladder cancer using EORTC risk tables: a combined analysis of 2596 patients from seven EORTC trials. Eur Urol 49:466–477; discussion 475–477

27. Yorukoglu K, Tuna B, Dikicioglu E et al (2003) Reproducibility of the 1998 World Health Organization/International Society of Urologic Pathology classification of papillary urothelial neoplasms of the urinary bladder. Virchows Arch 443:734–740

28. Schned AR, Andrew AS, Marsit CJ et al (2007) Survival following the diagnosis of noninvasive bladder cancer: WHO/International Society of Urological Pathology versus WHO classification systems. J Urol 178:1196–1200

29. Murphy WM, Takezawa K, Maruniak NA (2002) Interobserver discrepancy using the 1998 World Health Organization/International Society of Urologic Pathology classification of urothelial neoplasms: practical choices for patient care. J Urol 168:968–972

30. Bol MG, Baak JP, Buhr-Wildhagen S et al (2003) Reproducibility and prognostic variability of grade and lamina propria invasion in stages Ta, T1 urothelial carcinoma of the bladder. J Urol 169:1291–1294

31. Engers R (2007) Reproducibility and reliability of tumor grading in urological neoplasms. World J Urol 25:595–605

32. May M, Brookman-Amissah S, Roigas J et al (2010) Prognostic accuracy of individual uropathologists in noninvasive urinary bladder carcinoma: a multicentre study comparing the 1973 and 2004 World Health Organisation classifications. Eur Urol 57:850–858

33. van Rhijn BW, van Leenders GJ, Ooms BC et al (2010) The pathologist's mean grade is constant and individualizes the prognostic value of bladder cancer grading. Eur Urol 57:1052–1057

34. Gonul II, Poyraz A, Unsal C et al (2007) Comparison of 1998 WHO/ISUP and 1973 WHO classifications for interobserver variability in grading of papillary urothelial neoplasms of the bladder. Pathological evaluation of 258 cases. Urol Int 78:338–344

35. Cheng L, Lopez-Beltran A, MacLennan GT et al (2008) Neoplasms of the urinary bladder. In: Bostwick DG, Cheng L (eds) Urologic surgical pathology. Elsevier/Mosby, Philadelphia, pp 259–352

36. Cheng L, Montironi R, Davidson DD et al (2009) Staging and reporting of urothelial carcinoma of the urinary bladder. Mod Pathol 22(Suppl 2):S70–S95

37. Hofmann T, Knuchel-Clarke R, Hartmann A et al (2006) Clinical implications of the 2004 WHO histological classification on non-invasive tumours of the urinary bladder. EAUEBU 4:83–95

38. Cheng L, MacLennan GT, Lopez-Beltran A (2012) Histologic grading of urothelial carcinoma: a reappraisal. Hum Pathol 43:2097–2108

39. Mostofi FK, Sobin LH, Torloni H (1973) Histological typing of urinary bladder tumours. World Health Organization, Geneva

40. Cheng L, Darson M, Cheville JC et al (1999) Urothelial papilloma of the bladder: clinical and biologic implications. Cancer 86:2098–2101

41. Malmstrom PU, Bush C, Norlen BJ (1987) Recurrence, progression, and survival in bladder cancer. A retrospective analysis of 232 patients with greater than or equal to 5-year follow-up. Scand J Urol Nephrol 21:185–195

42. Prout GR, Barton BA, Griffin PP et al (1992) Treated history of noninvasive grade 1 transitional cell carcinoma. The National Bladder Cancer Group. J Urol 148:1413–1419

43. Holmang S, Hedelin H, Anderstrom C et al (1995) The relationship among multiple recurrences, progression and prognosis of patients with stages Ta and T1 transitional cell cancer of the bladder followed for at least 20 years. J Urol 153:1823–1827

44. England HR, Paris AMI, Blandy JP (1981) The correlation of T1 bladder tumour history with prognosis and follow-up requirements. Br J Urol 53:593–597

45. Leblanc B, Duclos AJ, Benard F et al (1999) Long-term followup of initial Ta grade 1 transitional cell carcinoma of the bladder. J Urol 162:1946–1960

46. Pocock RD, Ponder BA, O'Sullivan JP et al (1982) Prognostic factors in non-infiltrating carcinoma of the bladder: a preliminary report. Br J Urol 54:711–715

47. Gilbert HA, Logan JL, Kagan AR et al (1978) The natural history of papillary transitional cell carcinoma of the bladder and its treatment in any unselected population on the basis of histologic grading. J Urol 119:488–492

48. Heney NM, Ahmed S, Flanagan MJ et al (1983) Superficial bladder cancer: progression and recurrence. J Urol 130:1083–1086

49. Fitzpatrick JM, West AB, Butler MR et al (1986) Superficial bladder tumors (stage pTa, grades 1 and 2): the importance of recurrence pattern following initial resection. J Urol 135:920–922

50. Prout GR, Bassil B, Griffin P (1986) The treated histories of patients with Ta grade 1 transitional-cell carcinoma of the bladder. Arch Surg 121:1463–1468

51. Hemstreet GP 3rd, Rollins S, Jones P et al (1991) Identification of a high risk subgroup of grade 1 transitional cell carcinoma using image analysis based deoxyribonucleic acid ploidy analysis of tumor tissue. J Urol 146:1525–1529

52. Mufti GR, Virdi JS, Singh M (1990) 'Solitary' Ta-T1 G1 bladder tumour–history and long-term prognosis. Eur Urol 18:101–106

53. Jordan AM, Weingarten J, Murphy WM (1987) Transitional cell neoplasms of the urinary bladder. Can biologic potential be predicted from histologic grading. Cancer 60:2766–2774

54. Fitzpatrick JM (1993) Superficial bladder carcinoma. World J Urol 11:142–147

55. Greene L, Hanash K, Farrow G (1973) Benign papilloma or papillary carcinoma of the bladder. J Urol 110:205–207

56. Bostwick DG (1992) Natural history of early bladder cancer. J Cell Biochem 161(Suppl):31–38

57. Pauwels RP, Schapers RF, Smeets AW et al (1988) Grading in superficial bladder cancer: morphological criteria. Br J Urol 61:129–134

58. Schapers RF, Pauwels RP, Wijnen JT et al (1994) A simplified grading method of transitional cell carcinoma of the urinary bladder: reproducibility, clinical

significance and comparison with other prognostic parameters. Br J Urol 73:625–631

59. Carbin B, Ekman P, Gustafson H et al (1991) Grading of human urothelial carcinoma based on nuclear atypia and mitotic frequency. I. Histological description. J Urol 145:968–971

60. Lipponen PK, Eskelinen MJ, Kiviranta J et al (1991) Prognosis of transitional cell bladder cancer: a multivariate prognostic score for improved prediction. J Urol 146:1535–1540

61. Bostwick DG, Lopez-Beltran A (1999) Bladder biopsy interpretation. United Pathologists Press, Washington DC

62. Eble JN, Sauter G, Epstein JI et al (2004) World Health Organization classification of tumours: pathology and genetics of tumours of the urinary system and male genital organs. IARC Press, Lyon

63. Alsheikh A, Mohamedali Z, Jones E et al (2001) Comparison of the WHO/ISUP classification and cytokeratin 20 expression in predicting the behavior of low-grade papillary urothelial tumors. World/Health Organization/International Society of Urologic Pathology. Mod Pathol 14:267–272

64. Alvarez KJ, Lopez-Beltran A, Anglada CF et al (2001) Clinico-pathologic differences between bladder neoplasm with low malignant potential and low-grade carcinoma. Actas Urol Esp 25:645–650

65. Montironi R, Lopez-Beltran A (2005) The 2004 WHO classification of bladder tumors: a summary and commentary. Int J Surg Pathol 13:143–153

66. Cheng L, Neumann RM, Bostwick DG (1999) Papillary urothelial neoplasms of low malignant potential. Clinical and biologic implications. Cancer 86:2102–2108

67. Pan CC, Chang YH, Chen KK et al (2010) Prognostic significance of the 2004 WHO/ISUP classification for prediction of recurrence, progression, and cancer-specific mortality of non-muscle-invasive urothelial tumors of the urinary bladder: a clinicopathologic study of 1,515 cases. Am J Clin Pathol 133:788–795

68. Samaratunga H, Makarov DV, Epstein JI (2002) Comparison of WHO/ISUP and WHO classification of noninvasive papillary urothelial neoplasms for risk of progression. Urology 60:315–319

69. Holmang S, Andius P, Hedelin H et al (2001) Stage progression in Ta papillary urothelial tumors: relationship to grade, immunohistochemical expression of tumor markers, mitotic frequency and DNA ploidy. J Urol 165:1124–1130

70. Lee TK, Chaux A, Karram S et al (2011) Papillary urothelial neoplasm of low malignant potential of the urinary bladder: clinicopathologic and outcome analysis from a single academic center. Hum Pathol 42:1799–1803

71. Oyasu R (2000) World Health Organization and International Society of Urological Pathology Classification and two-number grading system of bladder tumors. Cancer 88:1509–1512

72. Herr HW, Donat SM, Reuter VE (2007) Management of low grade papillary bladder tumors. J Urol 178:1201–1205

73. Miyamoto H, Brimo F, Schultz L et al (2010) Low-grade papillary urothelial carcinoma of the urinary bladder: a clinicopathologic analysis of a post-World Health Organization/International Society of Urological Pathology classification cohort from a single academic center. Arch Pathol Lab Med 134:1160–1163

74. Pellucchi F, Freschi M, Ibrahim B et al (2011) Clinical reliability of the 2004 WHO histological classification system compared with the 1973 WHO system for Ta primary bladder tumors. J Urol 186:2194–2199

75. Habuchi T, Ogawa O, Kakehi Y et al (1993) Accumulated allelic losses in the development of invasive urothelial cancer. Int J Cancer 53:5093–5095

76. Chaux A, Karram S, Miller JS et al (2012) High-grade papillary urothelial carcinoma of the urinary tract: a clinicopathologic analysis of a post-World Health Organization/International Society of Urological Pathology classification cohort from a single academic center. Hum Pathol 43:115–120

77. Whisnant RE, Bastacky SI, Ohori NP (2003) Cytologic diagnosis of low-grade papillary urothelial neoplasms (low malignant potential and low-grade carcinoma) in the context of the 1998 WHO/ISUP classification. Diagn Cytopathol 28:186–190

78. Bircan S, Candir O, Serel TA (2004) Comparison of WHO 1973, WHO/ISUP 1998, WHO 1999 grade and combined scoring systems in evaluation of bladder carcinoma. Urol Int 73:201–208

79. Yin H, Leong AS (2004) Histologic grading of noninvasive papillary urothelial tumors: validation of the 1998 WHO/ISUP system by immunophenotyping and follow-up. Am J Clin Pathol 121:679–687

80. Curry JL, Wojcik EM (2002) The effects of the current World Health Organization/International Society of Urologic Pathologists bladder neoplasm classification system on urine cytology results. Cancer 96:140–145

81. Ramos D, Navarro S, Villamon R, Gil-Salom M, Llombart-Bosch A (2003) Cytokeratin expression patterns in low-grade papillary urothelial neoplasms of the urinary bladder. Cancer 97:1876–1883

82. Burger M, Denzinger S, Wieland WF et al (2008) Does the current World Health Organization classification predict the outcome better in patients with noninvasive bladder cancer of early or regular onset? BJU Int 102:194–197

83. Campbell PA, Conrad RJ, Campbell CM et al (2004) Papillary urothelial neoplasm of low malignant potential: reliability of diagnosis and outcome. BJU Int 93:1228–1231

84. Desai S, Lim SD, Jimenez RE et al (2000) Relationship of cytokeratin 20 and CD44 protein expression with WHO/ISUP grade in pTa and pT1 papillary urothelial neoplasia. Mod Pathol 13:1315–1323

85. Cheng L, Neumann RM, Nehra A et al (2000) Cancer heterogeneity and its biologic implications in the grading of urothelial carcinoma. Cancer 88:1663–1670

86. Eble JN, Young RH (1989) Benign and low grade papillary lesions of the urinary bladder: a review of

the papilloma-papillary carcinoma controversy and a report of five typical papillomas. Semin Diagn Pathol 6:351–371

87. Epstein JI, Amin MB, Reuter VR et al (1998) The World Health Organization/International Society of Urological Pathology consensus classification of urothelial (transitional cell) neoplasms of the urinary bladder. Bladder Consensus Conference Committee. Am J Surg Pathol 22:1435–1448

88. Mostofi FK, Davis CJ, Sesterhenn IA (1999) WHO histologic typing of urinary bladder tumors. Springer, Berlin

89. Burger M, van der Aa MN, van Oers JM et al (2008) Prediction of progression of non-muscle-invasive bladder cancer by WHO 1973 and 2004 grading and by FGFR3 mutation status: a prospective study. Eur Urol 54:835–843

Tumors of the Prostate

9

Ming Zhou

9.1 Introduction

Carcinoma of the prostate (PCa) is the most common non-cutaneous malignancy in males. Needle biopsy, via transrectal or transperineal approach, is performed to establish the diagnosis of PCa. Grading of PCa has major clinical implications for planning the treatment and formulating the prognosis [1, 2].

The most widely used and best clinically tested system is the one developed by Dr. Donald Gleason [3, 4]. The system is relatively simple and reasonably reproducible. Although there is considerable interobserver variability, especially in needle biopsy specimens, the Gleason score is the most important prognostic factor in predicting findings in radical prostatectomy, biochemical failure, and local and distant metastasis in patients after therapy. It is also an integral part of multifactorial prognosis prediction models.

9.2 The Original Gleason Grading System

The Gleason grading system is based purely on the architectural pattern of PCa (Fig. 9.1a), using a scale from 1 to 5 [3, 4], which represents

M. Zhou, M.D., Ph.D.
Surgical Pathology and Urologic Pathology,
NYU Medical Center Tisch Hospital,
560 First Avenue, TCH-461,
New York, NY 10016-6497, USA
e-mail: ming.zhou@nyumc.org

increasing deviation from the morphology of normal prostate glands. The tumor is examined to determine the most and second most predominant patterns, which are designated as the *primary and secondary grades*. An innovative feature of this system is that the primary and secondary grades are added up and reported as the Gleason score.

9.3 2005 International Society of Urological Pathology (ISUP) Modified Gleason Grading System

Since the inception of Gleason grading system some 40 years ago, the Gleason grading system has remained as one of the most powerful prognostic indicators in PCa. One of the main reasons is that it has remained timely by continuous adaptation to changes in the diagnosis and clinical management of prostate cancer [5, 6]. However, some aspects of the original grading system are interpreted differently in contemporary pathology practice. With such changes have come variations in applying the Gleason grading system among practicing pathologists. Therefore, the International Society of Urological Pathology (ISUP) convened a conference in 2005 in an attempt to achieve consensus in controversial areas in Gleason grading of PCa [7]. It is important to stress that the changes put forth by 2005 ISUP modified Gleason grading system were not "invented" de novo, rather they have already been implemented in practice

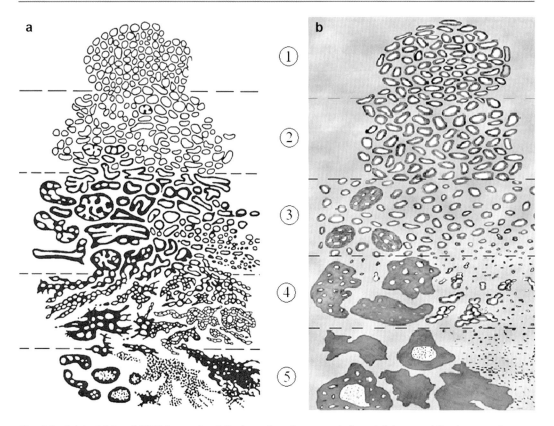

Fig. 9.1 Original (**a**) and 2005 International Society of Urological Pathology (ISUP) modified (**b**) Gleason grading system. Both grading schemes include five architectural patterns that represent an increasing deviation from the normal prostate glandular architecture. The definition of patterns 1, 2, and 5 is essentially the same between these two systems. However, cancer glands of pattern 3 in the modified system are discrete and well differentiated. Cribriform glands and single cells are not allowed in the modified system

by many pathologists, and the consensus simply codified these changes.

The original and 2005 ISUP modified Gleason grading systems are summarized in Fig. 9.1 and Table 9.1. The highlights of the latter are outlined below in the comments.

9.3.1 Comments Regarding Gleason Grading System

1. 2005 ISUP modified Gleason grading system refined the criteria for grade 3. Only discrete, well-formed cancer glands are considered to be grade 3. Poorly formed glands and single cells are not allowed in grade 3. As the result, the grade 3 scope is narrowed and the grade 4 scope is expanded.

2. A Gleason score of $1 + 1 = 2$ should not be rendered, regardless of the specimen type, with only rare exceptions.

3. Gleason scores 2–4 in needle biopsies should rarely be rendered in needle biopsies, if ever. Practically, Gleason score in needle biopsy starts from $3 + 3 = 6$.

4. Most cribriform patterns are diagnosed as grade 4. A recent study found that all cribriform cancer glands should be diagnosed as grade 4 [8].

5. PCa has several histological patterns, including pseudohyperplastic carcinoma, foamy gland carcinoma, and cancer with cytoplasmic vacuoles and glomeruloid architecture. In addition, several histological variants are described. Their histological features and corresponding Gleason grading are shown in Table 9.2.

Table 9.1 The five architectural patterns in the original and 2005 ISUP modified Gleason grading system

Gleason pattern	Original Gleason system	2005 ISUP modified Gleason system	Key difference
1	Circumscribed nodule of closely packed, but separate, uniform, round to oval, medium-sized acini (larger than pattern 3)	Same as the original system (Fig. 9.2a)	None
2	Similar to pattern 1, fairly circumscribed, but at the edge of the tumor nodule, there may be minimal infiltration; glands more loosely arranged and not as uniform as pattern 1	Same as the original system (Fig. 9.2b)	Cribriform glands not allowed in the modified system
3	Similar to pattern 2 but marked irregularity in size and shape of cancer glands, with tiny glands or individual cells invading stroma away from circumscribed masses or solid cords and masses with easily identifiable glandular differentiation in majority of them	Discrete glandular units typically smaller than those in patterns 1 and 2 with marked variation in size and shape, infiltrating between noncancerous glands (Fig. 9.2c)	Poorly formed glands or individual cells not allowed in the modified system
4	Large clear cells growing in a diffuse pattern resembling clear cell renal carcinoma (hypernephroma) may show glandular formation	Ill-defined glands with poorly formed glandular lumina (Fig. 9.2d), fused microacinar glands (Fig. 9.2e), any cribriform glands (Fig. 9.2f), and hypernephromatoid pattern (Fig. 9.2g)	Cribriform glands and ill-defined glands with poorly formed lumina are pattern 4 in the modified system
5	Very poorly differentiated, usually solid masses or diffuse growth with little or no glandular differentiation	Essentially no glandular differentiation, with solid sheets (Fig. 9.2h), cords or single cells (Fig. 9.2i), and comedonecrosis in any architectural pattern (Fig. 9.2j)	No major difference

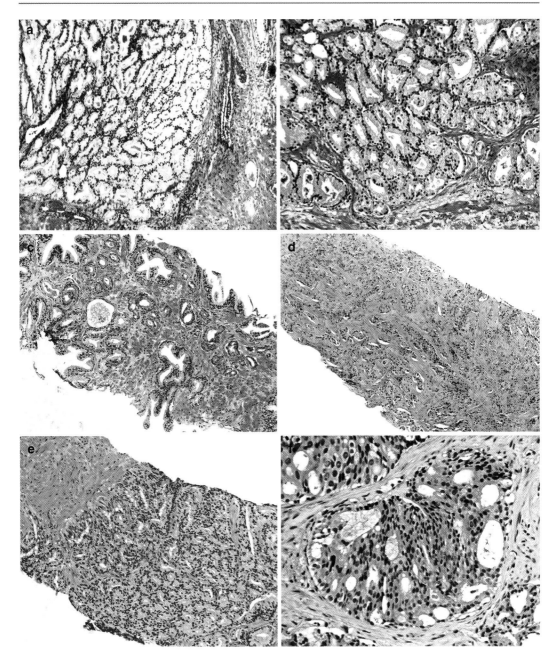

Fig. 9.2 2005 *International Society of Urological Pathology* (ISUP) modified Gleason grading system. (**a**) Pattern 1: The tumor is composed of uniform round glands closely packed into nodule that has well-defined margins and pushing borders. The tumor and stroma interface is smooth. The glands are medium sized and uniform. In between the glands, a distinct stroma is recognizable. This pattern is very rare and should not be diagnosed in needle biopsies. (**b**) Pattern 2: The tumor comprises round glands that show more variation in size and shape and are less evenly spaced than in Gleason pattern 1 tumors. The tumor nodules do not have round contours and appear incompletely circumscribed. The stroma is more abundant. This pattern should not, or rarely, be rendered in prostate biopsy. (**c**) Pattern 3: The tumor is composed of neoplastic glands of variable sizes, shape, and spacing infiltrating between benign glands. The acini are discrete and separated from each other by strands of fibrous stroma. The glands are well formed, with easily discernible lumens. (**d–g**) Pattern 4: Cancer glands may present in several architectural forms, including ill-defined glands with poorly formed glandular lumina (**d**), fused glands (**e**), cribriform glands (**f**), and hypernephromatoid pattern (**g**). (**h–j**) Pattern 5: Cancer glands essentially exhibit no glandular differentiation, with solid sheets (**h**), cords or single cells (**i**), and comedonecrosis in any architectural pattern (**j**)

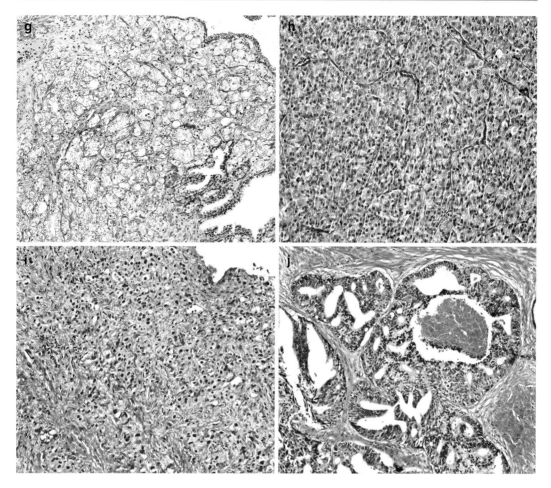

Fig. 9.2 (continued)

9.3.2 Specific Issues Regarding Prostate Needle Biopsies

1. In needle biopsy, high-grade tumor (grade 4 and 5) of any quantity should be included and reported in the final Gleason score. For example, if a PCa contains 98 % grade 3 component and 2 % grade 5 component in needle biopsy, the Gleason score should be $3+5=8$.
2. Secondary patterns of lower-grade cancer, when present to a limited extent (<5 %) in the setting of a high-grade cancer, should be ignored and not reported.
3. If a biopsy contains multiple patterns with 3, 4, and 5 in various proportions and pattern 5 being the least (tertiary pattern), the final grade should include pattern 5 as the secondary pattern.
4. For biopsies with different cores showing different grades, each core should be assigned an individual grade if they are submitted in separate containers or their anatomic site is specified by urologists (by different inking) even when they are submitted in the same container. An overall or global Gleason score may be provided. When multiple cores are put in a container without site specification and more than one core contain PCa, some pathologists grade each core separately, while others would only provide an overall Gleason score. If, however, the cores are fragmented, an overall score should be given.

Table 9.2 Gleason grading of histological variants and patterns of prostate carcinoma

Histology	Histological feature	Gleason grading
Histological patterns		
Glomeruloid body	Balls of tufts of cancer cells within glands	3 or 4, recent data suggest grade 4
Collagenous micronodule	Acellular or hypocellular hyalinized stroma within or outside cancer glands	Based on the underlying glandular architecture
Foamy gland	Cancer cells with abundant foamy cytoplasm	Based on the underlying glandular architecture
Pseudohyperplastic	Many closely packed glands of varying size with complex and undulating architecture and frequent papillary infolding	Grade 3
Atrophic	Cancer cells with reduced cytoplasm	Grade 3
Intracytoplasmic vacuoles	Clear vacuoles within the cytoplasm of cancer cells	Based on the underlying glandular architecture
Histological variants		
Ductal carcinoma	Papillary, cribriform, or solid growth pattern with glands lined with stratified columnar-shaped nuclei	Grade 4; grade 5 if solid and comedonecrosis is present
High-grade PIN-like	Large crowded cancer glands with irregular contour, resembling high-grade PIN	Grade 3
Mucinous	Caner glands with abundant extravasated mucin, accounting for >25 % of tumor volume	Based on the glandular architecture
Neuroendocrine differentiation	Paneth-like cells or cells positive for neuroendocrine markers	Paneth-like cells or cells positive for neuroendocrine markers are not considered to have prognostic significance, therefore do not change the Gleason grade
	Small-cell carcinoma	Small-cell carcinoma not graded
Signet-ring cell carcinoma	Single cells with cytoplasmic vacuoles	Grade 5
Pleomorphic giant cell	Pleomorphic and giant cancer cells, usually with known history of PCa with treatment; positive for prostate markers	Grade 4 or 5, not graded if after treatment
Sarcomatoid	Malignant spindle cells or specific soft tissue differentiation	Not graded
Adenosquamous and squamous carcinoma	Malignant squamous component with or without glandular component	Not graded

9.3.3 Specific Issues Regarding Radical Prostatectomy Specimens

1. Tertiary pattern. Gleason score should be obtained by adding the primary and secondary grades together. However, a tertiary pattern higher than the primary and secondary grades should be included in the final Gleason score as the secondary grade when it is >5 % of the tumor. It can be reported as tertiary pattern if it is <5 % of the tumor.

2. Radical prostatectomy with separate tumor nodules. Not uncommonly, a radical prostatectomy specimen contains several tumor nodules of significant sizes.

Gleason scores should be rendered to each tumor nodule if they are of different grades. Most often, the dominant nodule is the largest tumor and is associated with the highest stage and highest grade. Rarely, a nondominant nodule (i.e., smaller nodule) has a higher stage; one should also assign a grade to that nodule.

Books and Monographs

Amin MB, Grignon DJ, Humphrey PA, Srigley JR (2004) Gleason grading of prostate cancer: a contemporary approach. Lippincott Williams & Wilkins, Philadelphia

Bostwick DG, Cheng L (2008) Urologic surgical pathology, 2nd edn. Mosby/Elsevier, Edinburgh

Eble JN, Sauter G, Epstein JE, Sesterhenn IA (eds) (2004) World Health Organization classification of tumors: pathology and genetics. Tumours of the urinary system and male genital organs. IARC Press, Lyon

Articles

1. Epstein JI (2010) An update of the Gleason grading system. J Urol 183:433–440
2. Gleason DF (1992) Histologic grading of prostate cancer: a perspective. Hum Pathol 23:273–279
3. Gleason DF, Mellinger GT (1974) Prediction of prognosis for prostatic adenocarcinoma by combined histological grading and clinical staging. J Urol 111:58–64
4. Mellinger GT, Gleason D, Bailar J 3rd (1967) The histology and prognosis of prostatic cancer. J Urol 97:331–337
5. Egevad L, Mazzucchelli R, Montironi R (2012) Implications of the International Society of Urological Pathology modified Gleason grading system. Arch Pathol Lab Med 136:426–434
6. Lotan TL, Epstein JI (2010) Clinical implications of changing definitions within the Gleason grading system. Nat Rev Urol 7:136–142
7. Epstein JI, Allsbrook WC Jr, Amin MB et al (2005) The 2005 International Society of Urological Pathology (ISUP) consensus conference on Gleason grading of prostatic carcinoma. Am J Surg Pathol 29:1228–1242
8. Latour M, Amin MB, Billis A et al (2008) Grading of invasive cribriform carcinoma on prostate needle biopsy: an interobserver study among experts in genitourinary pathology. Am J Surg Pathol 32:1532–1539

Tumors of the Female Genital Organs

10

Jaime Prat and Ivan Damjanov

10.1 Introduction

Tumors of the female genital organs are often biopsied or surgically resected and thus form a significant part of surgical pathology material in most institutions. Invasive tumors and premalignant or borderline lesions are routinely graded, and in many instances, the grade assigned by the pathologist is an important determinant of future treatment of these conditions. The parts of the female genital organs that are covered with squamous epithelium, namely, the vulva, vagina, and the cervix uteri, give rise to squamous cell carcinomas. Squamous cell carcinomas and their precursors of the female genital organs are graded like the homonymous lesions in other anatomic sites. The mucosa of the endocervix, endometrium, fallopian tubes, and probably the surface epithelium (mesothelium) of the ovary give rise to adenocarcinomas. These tumors are graded more or less the same way as adenocarcinomas in other anatomic locations. Some ovarian tumors that are unique to that organ are graded according to generally accepted schemes.

J. Prat, M.D., Ph.D., FRCPath (✉)
Department of Pathology, Hospital de la Santa Creu i Sant Pau, Autonomous University of Barcelona, Sant Quintí, 87-89, Barcelona, Spain
e-mail: jprat@santpau.cat

I. Damjanov, M.D., Ph.D.
Department of Pathology,
The University of Kansas School of Medicine,
Kansas City, KS, USA
e-mail: idamjano@kumc.edu

10.2 Vulvar Squamous Intraepithelial Neoplasia

Keratinizing squamous cell carcinoma of the vulva is preceded by intraepithelial changes [1]. These changes can be recognized microscopically as vulvar squamous intraepithelial neoplasia (VIN), well differentiated, or simplex (Fig. 10.1). VIN originating in the context of long-standing lichen sclerosus carries a high risk of cancer development. In contrast, the less common HPV-associated basaloid and warty carcinomas develop from a precursor lesion called undifferentiated or classic VIN (Fig. 10.2). HPV-associated VIN lesions have a low risk of progression to invasive carcinomas (approximately 6 %), except in older or immunosuppressed women.

10.2.1 Well-Differentiated (Simplex) VIN

In this form of VIN, the nuclear atypia is confined to the basal and parabasal layer (Fig. 10.1a). The squamous cells show abundant eosinophilic cytoplasm and prominent intercellular bridges (Fig. 10.1b). The nuclei are relatively uniform in size and contain coarse chromatin and prominent nucleoli. Occasional pearls are seen. Until recently, well-differentiated VIN had been misinterpreted as squamous hyperplasia. Grading of this lesion is poorly reproducible. Most cases are VIN 3.

I. Damjanov, F. Fan (eds.), *Cancer Grading Manual*,
DOI 10.1007/978-3-642-34516-6_10, © Springer-Verlag Berlin Heidelberg 2013

Fig. 10.1 Vulvar intraepithelial neoplasia (*VIN*) well-differentiated (*simplex*) type. (**a**) The atypia is accentuated in the basal and parabasal layers. (**b**) There is striking epithelial maturation in the superficial layers. The keratinocytes show abundant eosinophilic cytoplasm and prominent intercellular bridges

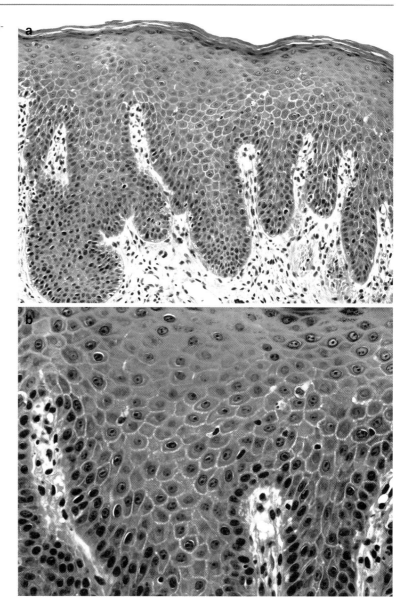

10.2.2 HPV-Related or Classic VIN

This form of VIN is graded according to the principles similar to those used in the grading of preinvasive neoplasia of the cervix, i.e., on a scale from 1 to 3, corresponding to mild, moderate, and severe dysplasia, respectively. However, grade 3—which includes squamous cell carcinoma in situ (CIS)—is by far the most common (Fig. 10.2).

- *VIN 1—mild squamous dysplasia*. The epithelium is slightly thickened and has a disorganized basal layer showing mild nuclear atypia.

In the superficial layers, there is prominent koilocytosis. The surface may be covered with a hyperkeratotic layer and an underlying layer of granular cells, resembling those in the skin (Fig. 10.2a).

- *VIN 2—moderate squamous dysplasia*. The epithelium shows disorganized layering, nuclear enlargement and irregularity, and mitotic activity in lower two-thirds of the squamous epithelium. Squamous maturation with proper layering is retained toward the surface (Fig. 10.2b).

Fig. 10.2 Vulvar intraepithelial neoplasia, classic type. (**a**) VIN1, the epithelium is thickened, slightly disorganized, and shows koilocytosis in the superficial layers. (**b**) VIN2, the thickened epithelium shows disorganized layering and contains cells that have enlarged, irregular, and hyperchromatic nuclei. Squamous maturation with proper layering is retained toward the surface. There is surface parakeratosis. (**c**) VIN3, the entire thickness of the epithelium contains hyperchromatic, small atypical basaloid cells. The surface shows hyperkeratosis or parakeratosis

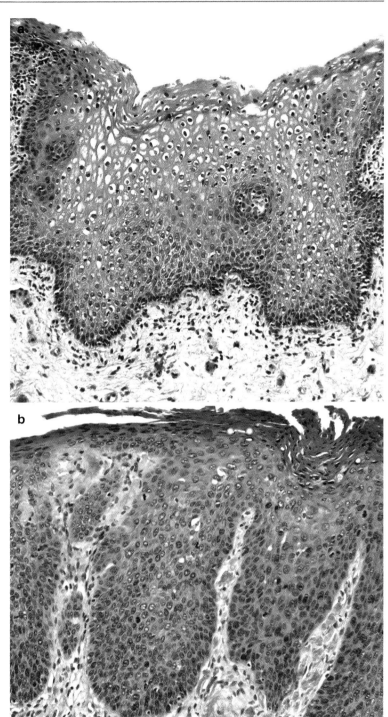

Fig. 10.2 (continued)

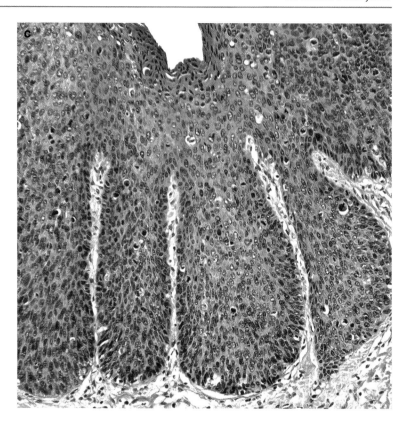

- *VIN 3—severe squamous dysplasia/carcinoma in situ.* In this condition, the epithelium is frequently thickened. The entire thickness of the epithelium has been replaced by small atypical hyperchromatic basaloid cells with numerous mitoses. A thin layer of parakeratosis or abortive layering may be seen on the surface (Fig. 10.2c). In some cases of VIN 3, there is prominent surface hyperkeratosis, and the entire lesion has a verrucous appearance (*warty type of VIN 3*). Bowen disease is a synonym for VIN III of the classic type.

10.3 Invasive Squamous Cell Carcinoma of the Vulva

Invasive squamous cell carcinoma of the vulva is graded according to the same principles as the squamous carcinoma in other anatomic locations.

- *Grade 1—well-differentiated squamous cell carcinoma.* Tumor cells resemble normal squamous epithelium with frequent formation of concentrically laminated keratin pearls. The tumor cells are polygonal and have well-developed eosinophilic cytoplasm. The intercellular bridges are seen clearly at high magnification. The nuclei show mild atypia with inconspicuous nucleoli. There are occasional mitoses.
- *Grade 2—moderately differentiated squamous cell carcinoma.* Tumor cells have variable amounts of cytoplasm and pleomorphic nuclei. Squamous differentiation of the tumor cells is still recognizable by occasional keratin pearls formation and individual cell keratinization. Mitoses are easily identified.
- *Grade 3—poorly differentiated squamous cell carcinoma.* Tumor cells have a high nuclear-cytoplasmic ratio and show nuclear hyperchromasia and pleomorphism. Individual cell keratinization may be seen, but no keratin pearls are found. In some tumors, the nests are composed of small basaloid cells that show almost no signs of squamous differentiation. Mitoses are prominent and often atypical.

Invasive squamous cell carcinoma may be also classified as keratinizing and nonkeratinizing. The keratinizing squamous cell carcinoma is usually well differentiated, whereas the nonkeratinizing squamous cell carcinomas are usually moderately to poorly differentiated. Several additional microscopic subtypes are recognized. These rare forms of carcinoma include the following:

- *Basaloid squamous cell carcinoma.* These tumors are composed of sheets of small, ovoid cells resembling those in HPV-related VIN 3. It tends to occur in younger women infected with HPV.
- *Sarcomatoid squamous cell carcinoma.* This is a poorly differentiated carcinoma and immunohistochemistry may be needed to distinguish it from sarcoma.
- *Verrucous squamous cell carcinoma.* This is a rare well-differentiated squamous cell carcinoma that forms papillary fronds and invades the underlying stroma forming bulbous pegs with a pushing border. It resembles condyloma acuminatum and is related to HPV infection.
- *Warty squamous cell carcinoma.* This is a rare exophytic tumor composed of papillae covered with a thick layer of parakeratosis and keratosis. It contains koilocytes, and it is typically associated with HPV infection.
- *Keratoacanthoma-like squamous cell carcinoma.* This low-grade tumor grows fast but does not invade or metastasize. Typically, it occurs on the hair-covered part of the vulva and is identical to keratoacanthoma-like squamous cell carcinomas on other parts of the skin.

10.3.1 Comments

1. Most of the vulvar and vaginal squamous cell carcinomas are moderately differentiated, whereas the well-differentiated and poorly differentiated squamous cell carcinomas occur less often.
2. The grade of tumors is directly related to the risk for lymph node metastasis and the overall poor prognosis.

3. Grading and staging are important prognostic predictors for vulvar squamous cell carcinomas. The number of inguinal lymph node metastases is the most important single factor. Only one-fourth of patients with pelvic node metastases live 5 years. Additional immunohistochemical studies do not seem to contribute significantly to the data obtained by thorough clinicopathologic work-up [2, 3].

10.4 Tumors of the Vagina

Tumors of the vagina are less common than those of the vulva or the cervix. Most of the tumors originate from the squamous epithelium. Glandular and mesenchymal tumors are rare.

Squamous cell neoplasms of the vagina, which account for over 95 % of all vaginal cancers, occur in an invasive and a preinvasive form. Preinvasive neoplasms are identical to intraepithelial squamous cell lesions of the vulva and cervix. These lesions are called vaginal intraepithelial neoplasm (VAIN) and are graded on scale from 1 to 3 as mild, moderate, or severe. Invasive tumors present as keratinizing or nonkeratinizing squamous cell carcinomas identical to those in the vulva or the cervix.

10.5 Cervical Intraepithelial Neoplasia

Essentially all squamous cell carcinomas of the cervix are preceded by cervical intraepithelial neoplasia (CIN) and are in most instances related to infection with human papilloma viruses [4, 5]. CIN can be diagnosed reliably by exfoliative cytology and in histologic sections of the cervical lesions.

CIN is graded on a scale from 1 to 3 or designated as mild, moderate, or severe squamous dysplasia. The rubric CIN 3 includes not only severe dysplasia but also carcinoma in situ of the cervix; these two lesions cannot be separated objectively one from another.

Intraepithelial lesions can be also graded in a binary system as low-grade squamous intraepithelial

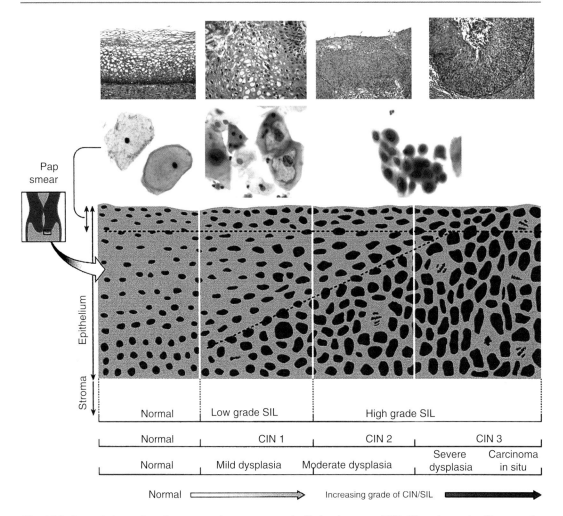

Fig. 10.3 Interrelations of naming systems in precursor cervical lesions. This chart integrates multiple aspects of the disease. It illustrates the changes in progressively more abnormal disease states and provides translation terminology for the dysplasia/carcinoma in situ (*CIS*) system, cervical intraepithelial neoplasia (*CIN*) system, and the Bethesda system (*SIL*). The scheme also illustrates the corresponding cytologic smear resulting from exfoliation of the most superficial cells as well as the equivalent histopathologic lesions (*top*). Abbreviation: *SIL* squamous intraepithelial lesion

lesions (LSIL) or high-grade squamous intraepithelial lesions (HSIL). The comparison of the three-tiered and the two-tiered grading system, the Bethesda cytologic system, and the HPV risk group is presented in Fig. 10.3.

Even though there is still some interobserver variation [6], the 3-tiered system of grading is currently the most widely used one. It includes the following categories:

- *CIN 1—mild squamous dysplasia*. This lesion results from HPV infection causing disorderly proliferation of cells in the lower third of the epithelium. These layers are widened and lack normal polarization, but are still distinct from the two surface layers which show layering and signs of squamous maturation. The cells have enlarged hyperchromatic nuclei. In the lower layers, nuclear enlargement results in a high nucleocytoplamic ratio. In upper layers, nuclear enlargement results in formation of koilocytes. Koilocytes have an optically clear cytoplasm and contain enlarged hyperchromatic nuclei of irregular contours ("raisinoid-nuclei"). These nuclei are eccentrically located and appear to be in contact with the cell membrane on one side. Mitoses may be seen but are confined to the basal layer and do not show morphologic atypia (Fig. 10.4a).

- *CIN 2—moderate squamous dysplasia.* This lesion shows marked cellular atypia and a loss of cellular polarity throughout the lower two-thirds of the epithelium. The upper third of epithelium shows good layering of cells and surface squamous maturation. Nuclear enlargement, atypia, and hyperchromasia are

prominent, but the mitoses are limited to the lower two-thirds of the epithelium. Abnormal mitotic figures may be present (Fig. 10.4b).

- *CIN 3—severe squamous dysplasia/carcinoma in situ.* The epithelium shows no signs of layering or maturation. From the bottom to the top, it is composed of atypical cells that have a high nucleocytoplasmic ratio. These basaloid cells (called so because they resemble normal basal cells) have spindle-shaped or irregularly shaped enlarged hyperchromatic nuclei

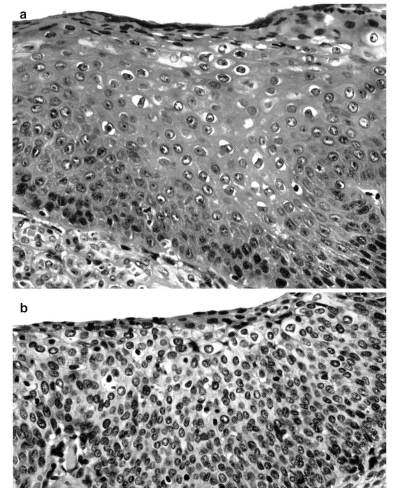

Fig. 10.4 (**a**) CIN 1, the epithelium is disorganized in the lower part but shows surface layering and koilocytosis. (**b**) CIN2, two-thirds of the entire thickness of the epithelium contain basaloid cells, but the upper third still shows layering and squamous differentiation. (**c**) CIN3, hyperchromatic small cells occupy the entire thickness of the epithelium, and there is almost no surface stratification or squamous differentiation

Fig. 10.4 (continued)

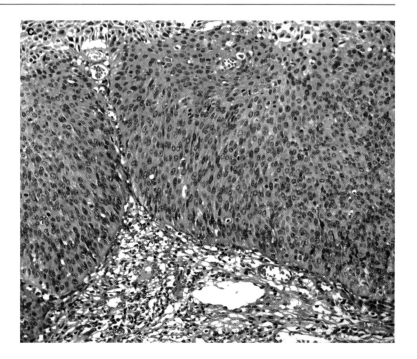

arranged disorderly and without any polarization. Mitotic figures are numerous and are found at random at all levels. The surface may show focal parakeratosis or hyperkeratosis. Abnormal mitoses are common (Fig. 10.4c).

10.5.1 Comments

1. CIN can involve foci of intraglandular squamous metaplasia in the endocervix. These changes must be distinguished from metaplasia and should not be mistaken for invasive carcinoma.
2. CIN 3 may be associated with microinvasive or overtly invasive squamous cell carcinomas. Even with modern technology available in the laboratory, it is difficult to predict which CIN will progress to invasive carcinoma [7].
3. The transition of CIN into invasive squamous cell carcinoma should be suspected in all cases of CIN that show the following features:
   - Involvement of broad areas of the cervix
   - Multifocal and deep extension into the glands of the endocervix
   - Marked thickening of the dysplastic epithelium and exophytic papillary growth pattern
   - Foci of squamous differentiation scattered at random and especially if found in the basal zones
   - Foci of surface necrosis of the dysplastic epithelium
   - Extensive chronic inflammation in the stroma underneath the dysplastic epithelium
4. Immunohistochemistry with antibody MIB-1 (Ki-67) shows high proliferative activity in all layers of CIN3. This is in sharp contrast to the normal epithelium and low-grade dysplasia in which MIB-1 reacts with nuclei of basal and parabasal layer only.

10.6 Invasive Squamous Cell Carcinoma of the Cervix

Invasive squamous cell carcinoma (SCC) is graded the same was as squamous cell carcinoma in other anatomic sites.
- *Grade 1—well-differentiated squamous cell carcinoma.* These tumors are composed of cells that resemble normal squamous epithelium with frequent formation of concentrically laminated keratin pearls and evident intercellular bridges. Tumor cells have abundant

Fig. 10.5 Invasive squamous cell carcinoma of the cervix. The tumor is composed of sheets of squamous cells that show individual keratinization

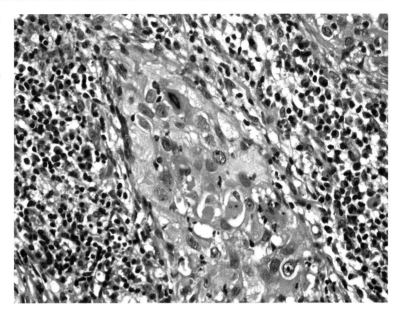

eosinophilic cytoplasm. Their nuclei show mild atypia with inconspicuous nucleoli and occasional mitosis.

- *Grade 2—moderately differentiated squamous cell carcinoma.* These tumors are composed of cells that have moderate amounts of cytoplasm and pleomorphic nuclei. Squamous differentiation of the tumor cells is still recognizable by occasional keratin pearls formation and individual cell keratinization. Mitoses are easily identified.
- *Grade 3—poorly differentiated squamous cell carcinoma.* These tumors are composed of cells that have a high nucleocytoplasmic ratio, marked nuclear pleomorphism, and abundant mitosis including some atypical forms. Individual keratinized cells may be seen (Fig. 10.5), but no keratin pearls formation is identified. Rarely, spindle-shaped tumor cells predominate resembling sarcoma.

Squamous cell carcinomas of the cervix are moderately differentiated in about two-thirds of all cases (Fig. 10.4), whereas the well-differentiated and poorly differentiated forms are less common. Several microscopic variants are recognized as follows:

- *Nonkeratinizing squamous cell carcinoma.* It is the most common form of cervical cancer accounting for 65 % of all cases. Most of them show only abortive squamous differentiation and are classified as moderately differentiated SCC.
- *Keratinizing squamous cell carcinoma.* These tumors show signs of squamous differentiation (intercellular bridges, keratohyaline granules, and dyskeratosis) and form keratin pearls. They are usually well- or moderately differentiated SCC.
- *Basaloid squamous cell carcinoma.* This is a high-grade and aggressive tumor composed of small hyperchromatic cells bearing some resemblance to basaloid cells in CIN3.
- *Papillary squamous cell carcinoma.* These tumors form papillae lined by epithelium that resembles CIN3 and also show focal invasion of the stroma. They show focal areas of squamous differentiation and are usually classified as moderately differentiated.
- *Verrucous squamous cell carcinoma.* These tumors are well differentiated and show prominent surface keratinization.
- *Lymphoepithelioma-like squamous cell carcinoma.* These tumors resemble those of the nasopharynx. They are composed of nests of poorly differentiated squamous cells intermixed with lymphocytes.

10.7 Adenocarcinoma of the Cervix

Invasive adenocarcinoma of the cervix is rarely associated with adenocarcinoma in situ. In contrast, squamous intraepithelial lesion (SIL) is found more frequently [8]. Invasive adenocarcinoma is graded as follows:

- *Grade 1—well-differentiated adenocarcinoma.* These neoplasms consist predominantly of glands, whereas the solid components form only 5 % of the entire tumor.
- *Grade 2—moderately differentiated adenocarcinoma.* These tumors consist of glands, but solid areas account for 5 % to less than 50 % of the tumor.
- *Grade 3—poorly differentiated adenocarcinoma.* These tumors are composed of poorly differentiated cells that form solid masses accounting for more than 50 % of the entire tumor mass.

In addition to adenocarcinomas that cannot be further classified (*adenocarcinoma, NOS*), several microscopic subtypes of endocervical carcinoma [9] are recognized as follows:

- *Mucinous adenocarcinoma.* These tumors may occur in several grades, i.e., as well-differentiated, moderately differentiated, and poorly differentiated adenocarcinomas. Most adenocarcinomas of the cervix are moderately differentiated and show little intracytoplasmic mucin; thus, the tumor glands resemble those of endometrioid carcinoma or exhibit a mixed endocervical and endometrioid appearance. This has led to confusion, with these tumors being regarded as endometrioid adenocarcinomas.
- Several variants of mucinous adenocarcinomas are recognized: minimal deviation adenocarcinoma and endocervical, intestinal, villoglandular, and signet ring variants of endocervical adenocarcinoma.
- *Endometrioid adenocarcinoma.* These tumors occur in several grades and resemble endometrioid carcinomas of the uterus. Immunohistochemically, adenocarcinomas that show strong positive immunoreaction for vimentin and ER and weak or negative immunostaining for p16[INK4A] are most likely of endometrial origin.

- *Clear cell adenocarcinoma.* These high-grade tumors consist of clear or hobnail-like cells arranged into solid areas and tubular glands or lining papillae. They resemble clear cell carcinomas of the ovary.
- *Serous adenocarcinoma.* These high-grade tumors resemble serous adenocarcinoma of the ovary. The diagnosis of primary serous carcinoma of the cervix should be made only after tumor spread from the ovary, fallopian tube, or endometrium has been excluded.
- *Mesonephric adenocarcinoma.* These tumors develop from mesonephric remnants in the lateral and posterior wall of the cervix. The tumor forms several glandular patterns, and dense eosinophilic material may be found in their lumen. They may be well, moderately, or poorly differentiated.
- *Adenosquamous carcinoma.* These are aggressive tumors and tend to metastasize more often than common adenocarcinomas or squamous cell carcinomas.
- *Adenoid cystic carcinoma.* These rare tumors are high-grade neoplasms similar to those developing more frequently in the salivary glands; however, unlike carcinomas of the salivary glands, the cervical tumors do not usually show perineural invasion and presents greater nuclear pleomorphism, high mitotic index, and necrosis. The stroma is typically composed of hyaline PAS-positive material of basement membrane type. This material represents the best histologic marker for cervical ACC. The immunostainings for basement membrane components, such as type IV collagen and laminin, are nearly always positive.

10.7.1 Comments

1. Adenocarcinoma (NOS) and mucinous carcinomas account for the vast majority of all endocervical cancers. The prognosis is mostly stage dependent, and the grading is of limited prognostic significance.
2. Early adenocarcinoma showing subtle invasiveness may be difficult to identify in

biopsy material. If the distance between neoplastic glands and thick-walled blood vessels is less than the thickness of the vessel wall, invasion should be suspected [10].

3. The distinction of endocervical adenocarcinomas from endometrial adenocarcinomas may be difficult. The presence of abundant intracellular mucin favors an endocervical origin, but most endometrial adenocarcinomas show focal mucinous differentiation, and some of them are largely mucinous. The stroma of the tumor may be helpful; in cervical tumors it is typically fibrous, whereas endometrial carcinomas usually contain very little stroma.

4. If a serous or clear cell carcinoma is identified in the cervix, it is important to first exclude a metastasis from an ovarian tumor before a diagnosis of a primary cervical tumor is made.

10.8 Adenocarcinoma of the Endometrium

Endometrial adenocarcinomas are the most common malignant tumors of the uterus. These tumors can be subdivided into two major groups:

- *Type I tumors.* This group comprises estrogen-related endometrioid carcinomas, which account for the majority (80 %) of endometrial carcinomas.
- *Type II tumors (nonendometrioid carcinomas).* Tumors of this group are unrelated to estrogen and occur more often in postmenopausal women. These tumors often resemble ovarian carcinomas and are mainly of serous and clear cell types [11, 12].

Whereas type II (nonendometrioid) carcinomas are considered high-grade tumors by definition and there is no need to grade them, grading of endometrioid carcinomas is prognostically very important. These tumors span the spectrum from very well differentiated to almost completely undifferentiated and probably merge at the higher end of the spectrum with nonendometrioid carcinomas.

10.8.1 Type I: Estrogen-Related ("Endometrioid") Adenocarcinomas

These tumors develop in women in the age group from 40 to 65 years, usually in the context of endometrial hyperplasia. The 2009 International Federation of Gynecology and Obstetrics (FIGO) grading system is based primarily upon architectural features [12, 13].

According to FIGO, *architectural grading* of endometrial adenocarcinoma takes into account the proportion of glandular and solid areas (Fig. 10.6). The tumors are graded as well differentiated (50 %), moderately differentiated (35 %), and poorly differentiated (15 %) as follows:

- *Grade 1—well-differentiated adenocarcinoma.* These tumors are composed of almost entirely of well-formed glands (Fig. 10.6a). Solid areas account for less than 5 % of the total mass. These tumors may contain foci of squamous epithelium or show so-called morular growth, but these should not be counted as solid areas. Solid growth is based only on the non-squamous (glandular) component.
- *Grade 2—moderately differentiated adenocarcinoma.* These tumors are also composed of well-formed glands, but also contain 6–50 % of solid areas (Fig. 10.6b). Like in grade 1 tumors, squamous and morular areas should not be taken into account when calculating the extent of solid areas.
- *Grade 3—poorly differentiated adenocarcinoma.* In these, the solid parts predominate forming more than 50 % of the tumor mass (Fig. 10.6c).

The presence of grade 3 nuclear features (i.e., marked nuclear pleomorphism, coarse chromatin, prominent nucleoli) in architecturally grade 1 or 2 tumors increases their grade by one. Most endometrioid carcinomas are architecturally grade 1, and assessment of whether the nuclear features are grade 3 is quite subjective. As previously stated, in serous carcinoma, clear cell carcinoma, and squamous cell carcinoma, nuclear grading takes precedence over architecture [12, 13].

Several variants of endometrioid adenocarcinoma are recognized which can also be graded according to FIGO [14]. These variants include the following:

- Variant with squamous differentiation
- Villoglandular variant
- Secretory variant
- Ciliated cell variant

10.8.2 Type II: Non-endometrioid Adenocarcinomas

These tumors are less common than endometrioid adenocarcinomas and usually develop in older women and in the background of endometrial atrophy. This group includes the following tumor types:

- *Serous adenocarcinomas.* These tumors are of high grade (Fig. 10.7).
- *Clear cell adenocarcinomas.* These tumors are of high grade.
- *Squamous cell carcinomas.* The grade of these tumors varies.
- *Transitional cell carcinomas.* These tumors are usually grade 2 and 3.
- *Small cell carcinomas.* These are high-grade tumors resembling oat cell carcinoma of the lung.

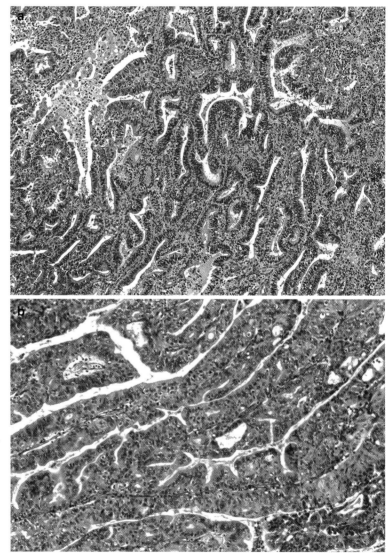

Fig. 10.6 Endometrioid adenocarcinoma of endometrium. (**a**) Grade 1, well-differentiated adenocarcinoma is composed of cells forming glands. (**b**) Grade 2, moderately differentiated adenocarcinoma consists of solid and glandular areas. (**c**) Grade 3, poorly differentiated adenocarcinoma consists mostly of solid sheets of cells

Fig. 10.6   (continued)

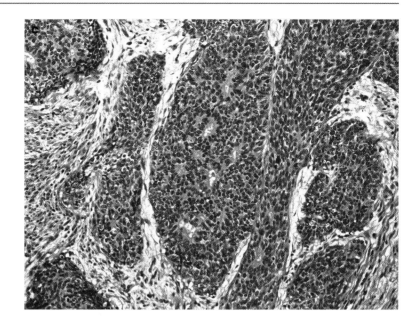

Fig. 10.7   Serous (*nonendo-metrioid*) adenocarcinoma of endometrium. There is stratification of anaplastic tumor cells (grade 3) showing prominent nucleoli and numerous mitoses

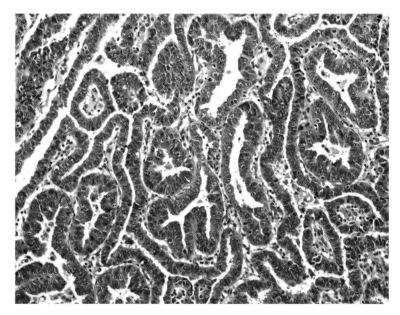

- *Undifferentiated carcinomas*. These are high-grade tumors.
- *Mucinous carcinomas*. These rare tumors tend to be low grade and therefore have an excellent prognosis.

10.8.3 Comments

1. The nuclear grades and the architectural grades of endometrioid adenocarcinomas usually correspond one to another. In the presence of marked nuclear atypia and the presence of bizarre nuclei, one should raise the architectural FIGO grade of grade 1 tumors to 2 and grade 2 tumors to 3.
2. Adenocarcinomas with squamous differentiation are graded according to the nuclear grade of the glandular component.
3. In serous adenocarcinomas, clear cell adenocarcinomas, and squamous cell carcinomas, nuclear grade takes precedence over the architectural grade.

4. Mixed adenocarcinoma is a term used for tumors that contain both type I endometrioid and type II nonendometrioid adenocarcinoma. The minor component must exceed 10 % of the total tumor mass. The tumors containing more than 25 % of type II tumors have a poor prognosis [14].

10.9   Smooth Muscle Tumors

Smooth muscle tumors may be divided into three groups: benign (leiomyomas), malignant (leiomyosarcomas), and tumors of unknown malignant potential (STUMP) [15, 16].

Leiomyoma. This is the most common benign uterine tumor. It is composed of smooth muscle cells and fibroblasts (Fig. 10.8a). Microscopically, the tumors are composed of fascicles of uniform spindle cells with elongated, blunt-ended nuclei, fine chromatin, small nucleoli, and eosinophilic abundant cytoplasm. Mitoses are infrequent (usually less than 5 per 10 high-power fields (hpf)). Hemorrhage, edema, myxoid degeneration, and hyaline fibrosis are common.

Several variants of leiomyoma are recognized. The most important that could be mistaken for leiomyosarcoma are:

- *Cellular leiomyoma.* This variant is characterized by prominent cellularity when compared to the surrounding myometrium. However, there is no coagulative tumor necrosis and no nuclear atypia or mitotic activity, which allows one to distinguish these tumors from leiomyosarcoma.
- *Mitotically active leiomyoma.* This variant has all the cellular and architectural features of typical leiomyomas but, at the same time, shows an increased mitotic activity (≥5 per 10). This diagnosis should be limited to tumors that show no significant marked nuclear atypia, contain no atypical mitosis, and no coagulative necrosis.
- *Atypical leiomyoma.* These tumors also known as symplastic, pleomorphic, or bizarre leiomyomas show marked nuclear atypia and intranuclear inclusions of cytoplasm. However, these nuclear changes are not associated with other features of malignancy of smooth muscle cell tumors. Thus, they show low mitotic activity (less than ten mitoses per 10 hpf) and lack areas of coagulative tumor cell necrosis [17].

- *Smooth muscle tumor of uncertain malignant potential (STUMP).* This term is used for tumors that cannot be histologically diagnosed with certainty as benign or malignant [15]. In general, STUMPs differ from leiomyomas and have some but not all features of leiomyosarcomas. The uterine smooth muscle tumors are diagnosed as STUMPs when they have the following features:
  - Coagulative necrosis present, but there is no increased mitotic activity and the nuclear atypia is not diffuse.
  - Increased mitotic activity (up to 15 mitoses per 10 hpf) is combined with focal atypia, but there is no diffuse atypia or any evidence of necrosis.
  - There is diffuse atypia, but there is no increased mitotic activity or any evidence of coagulative necrosis.

Leiomyosarcoma. This is a rare tumor, but nevertheless it represents the most common uterine sarcoma. The histopathologic diagnosis of uterine leiomyosarcoma is usually straightforward since most clinically malignant tumors show hypercellularity, severe nuclear atypia, and high mitotic rate generally exceeding 15 mitotic figures per 10 high-power fields (MF/10 hpf) (Fig. 10.8b). Moreover, large size (over 10 cm), infiltrating border, necrosis, and atypical mitotic figures are frequently present [16].

The minimal pathological criteria for the diagnosis of leiomyosarcoma are more problematic, and in such cases, the following combination of features supports the diagnosis:

- Coagulative necrosis and more than 10 mitoses per 10 hpf, with or without nuclear atypia.
- Coagulative necrosis, 10 or fewer than 10 mitoses per hpf with moderate to severe nuclear atypia.

No evidence of necrosis, but more than 10 mitoses per 10 hpf and diffuse moderate to severe nuclear atypia [15].

Fig. 10.8 Smooth muscle tumors of the uterus.
(**a**) Leiomyoma is composed of uniform smooth muscle cells and fibroblasts.
(**b**) Leiomyosarcoma contains hyperchromatic cells showing nuclear pleomorphism. Mitotic figures are numerous

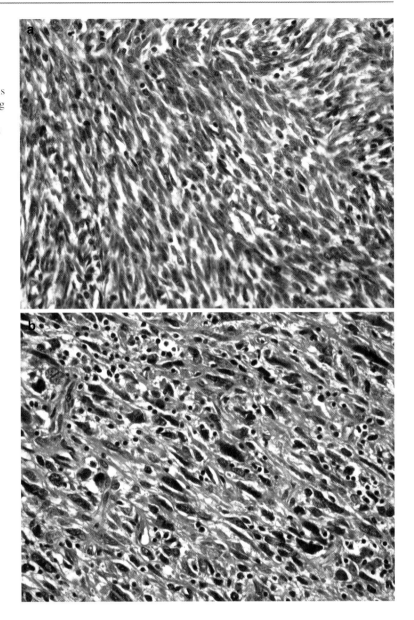

Epithelioid and myxoid leiomyosarcomas, however, are two rare variants which may be difficult to recognize microscopically as their pathologic features differ from those of ordinary spindle cell leiomyosarcomas. In fact, nuclear atypia is usually mild in both tumor types, and the mitotic rate is often <3 mitoses per 10 hpf. In epithelioid leiomyosarcomas, necrosis may be absent and myxoid leiomyosarcomas are often hypocellular. In the absence of severe cytologic atypia and high mitotic activity, both tumors are diagnosed as sarcomas based on their infiltrative borders [16].

Most uterine sarcomas are leiomyosarcomas. Exclusion of several histologic variants of leiomyoma, as well as STUMPs frequently misdiagnosed as sarcomas, has made apparent that the vast majority of leiomyosarcomas are high-grade sarcomas associated with poor prognosis even when confined to the uterus.

10.10 Adenocarcinoma of the Fallopian Tube

Adenocarcinomas of the fallopian tube are rare tumors. Morphologically they have the same features as endometrial or ovarian carcinomas and are graded according to the same principles [18].

10.11 Adenocarcinomas of the Ovary

Epithelial ovarian tumors are heterogeneous neoplasms which are primarily classified according to cell type into serous, mucinous, endometrioid, clear cell, transitional, and squamous cell tumors. Depending upon the degree of cell proliferation and nuclear atypia, and the presence or absence of stromal invasion, these tumors are further subdivided into benign, borderline (intermediate), and malignant (adenocarcinomas), and this subdivision correlates with prognosis. Adenocarcinomas of the ovary are the most common ovarian cancers accounting for 90 % of cases [19]. There are five main histologic types which by order of frequency are high-grade serous carcinomas (HGSC) (70 %), endometrioid carcinomas (EC) (10 %), clear cell carcinomas (CCC) (10 %), mucinous carcinomas (MC) (3 %), and low-grade serous carcinomas (LGSC) (<5 %) (Fig. 10.9). These tumors account for 98 % of ovarian adenocarcinomas and show different histopathological features, immunohistochemical profiles, and molecular genetic alterations.

It is now accepted that high-grade serous carcinoma (HGSC) and low-grade serous carcinoma (LGSC) are fundamentally different tumor types, and consequently different diseases. LGSC are associated in most cases with a serous borderline component, carry KRAS and BRAF mutations, and are unrelated to TP53 mutations and BRCA abnormalities. In contrast, HGSCs are not associated with serous borderline tumors and typically exhibit TP53 mutations and BRCA abnormalities [19].

Microscopically, HGSC shows papillary and solid growth with slit-like glandular lumens. The tumor cells are typically of intermediate size, with scattered bizarre mononuclear giant cells exhibiting prominent nucleoli (Fig. 10.9a). In contrast to LGSCs (Fig. 10.9b), these tumors show more than threefold variation in nuclear size. Although nuclear features are the chief criterion for distinguishing between HGSC and LGSC, the mitotic activity can be used in cases with equivocal degrees of nuclear pleomorphism; mitotic activity greater than 12/10 hpf favors a diagnosis of HGSC. In these tumors, mitotic activity is often several times this diagnostic threshold and is associated with abundant apoptotic bodies. High-grade and predominantly solid carcinomas showing serous differentiation, even in a minority of the tumor, should be classified as HGSC (rather than mixed serous/undifferentiated); to date, no underlying molecular differences between these tumors and pure HGSC have been detected [19]. Tumors showing nuclei of intermediate size often have TP53 mutations and should be classified as HGSC [20]. LGSC rarely progresses to high-grade tumors [19].

Mucinous adenocarcinomas (MC) of the ovary are often heterogeneous. Benign-appearing, borderline, noninvasive carcinoma, and invasive components may coexist within an individual tumor and suggest tumor progression from benign to borderline and from borderline to carcinoma. Therefore, extensive sampling for histological examination is necessary.

Recently, MCs have been divided into two categories: (a) an expansile type without obvious stromal invasion, but exhibiting back-to-back or complex malignant glands with minimal or no intervening stroma and exceeding 10 sq. mm in area (>3 mm in each of two linear dimensions) (Fig. 10.9c); and (b) an infiltrative type, showing evident stromal invasion in the form of glands, cell clusters, or individual cells, disorderly infiltrating the stroma and frequently associated with a desmoplastic stromal reaction [21, 22]. The expansile pattern of growth has also been referred to as the "noninvasive," "intraglandular," or "confluent glandular" pattern and is associated with a more favorable prognosis than the infiltrative pattern. A histopathological feature unique to mucinous tumors is the occasional finding of mural nodules of anaplastic carcinoma or high-grade sarcoma. When such nodules are localized in the wall of an unruptured cyst, the prognosis may be favorable, but such tumors may recur and do so as the anaplastic component [22, 23].

Endometrioid tumors of the ovary closely mimic their uterine counterparts. Most endometrioid carcinomas (EC) are low-grade adenocarcinomas and seem to arise from endometriotic cysts (Fig. 10.9d).

The architectural grade according to FIGO is assigned to EC as follows:

- *Grade 1—well-differentiated adenocarcinoma*. These tumors are composed predominantly of glands, with solid areas forming less than 5 % of the total tumor mass.
- *Grade 2—well-differentiated adenocarcinoma*. These tumors are composed of glands, but contain prominent solid areas occupying 6–50 % of the total tumor mass.
- *Grade 3—poorly differentiated adenocarcinoma*. In these tumors, the solid areas

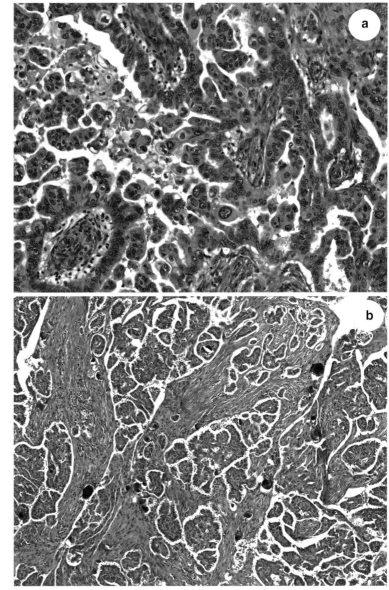

Fig. 10.9 Representative examples of the five main types of ovarian carcinoma, which together account for 98 % of cases: (**a**) High-grade serous carcinoma, (**b**) Low-grade serous carcinoma, (**c**) Mucinous carcinoma, (**d**) Endometrioid carcinoma, and (**e**) Clear cell carcinoma

Fig. 10.9 (continued)

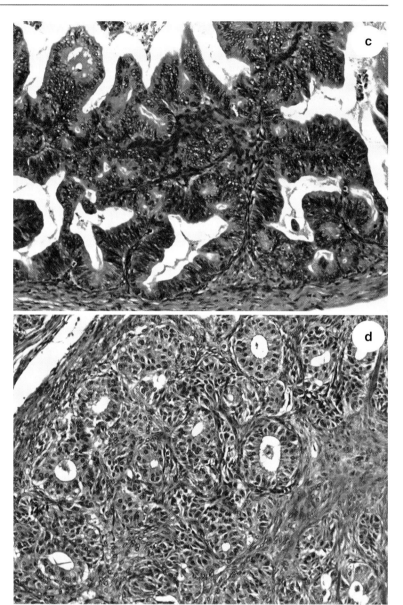

Fig. 10.9 (continued)

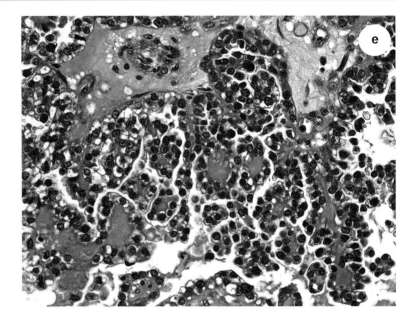

predominate forming more than 50 % of the tumor mass.

High-grade ECs are morphologically indistinguishable from HGSCs and often express Wilms' tumor gene (WT1). Gene expression profiling is also similar, suggesting that high-grade EC is not a distinct tumor type [19].

The presence of clear cells alone is not sufficient for a diagnosis of clear cell adenocarcinoma (CCC), as cells with clear cytoplasm can be seen in HGSC and EC. Besides the characteristic clear or hobnail cells with eccentric, rounded, and bulbous nuclei, the diagnosis is based on the following architectural and cytological findings: (a) multiple complex papillae, (b) densely hyaline basement membrane material expanding the cores of the papillae (Fig. 10.9e), and (c) hyaline bodies, which are present in approximately 25 % of cases. Mitoses are less frequent than in other types of ovarian carcinomas (usually less than 5/10 hpf). The vast majority of CCC are grade 3 tumors.

10.12   Germ Cell Tumors

Ovarian germ cell tumors are classified as benign or malignant. Teratoma, the most common benign germ cell tumor, is also the most common germ cell tumor in general accounting for over 90 % of tumors in this group. Secondary malignancy can occur in teratomas that have not been removed and were allowed to stay in the body until the woman reaches older age. Such malignant tumors are rare and are classified as squamous cell carcinoma, adenocarcinoma, neuroectodermal tumors, or sarcomas. Primary malignant germ cell tumors are also uncommon and include dysgerminoma, embryonal carcinoma, yolk sac tumor, and choriocarcinoma. Except for dysgerminoma, all other primary germ cell tumors are high-grade malignancies and are not graded.

Immature teratoma is the only germ cell tumor that is worth grading. Like the classical teratomas, these tumors contain various mature somatic tissues but also contain immature tissues most notably in the form of neuroectodermal tubes and rosettes [24]. Immature teratomas are graded on a scale from 1 to 3 as follows:

- *Grade 1 tumors.* These tumors contain only rare foci of immature neuroepithelial tissue occupying less than one low-power field in any slide.
- *Grade 2 tumors.* These tumors contain more immature neuroepithelial tissues, which occupy more than one but less than four low-power fields.
- *Grade 3 tumors.* These tumors contain abundant neuroepithelial elements occupying more than four low-power fields in any slide.

10.12.1 Comments

1. Immature ovarian teratomas may be associated with peritoneal glial nodules. These nodules do not represent metastases of the ovarian tumor, yet they should be also graded microscopically.
2. Multiple sections of the primary tumor and the peritoneal nodules must be submitted for proper grading.

10.13 Sex Cord: Stromal Tumors

Sex cord-stromal tumors account for less than 10 % of all ovarian tumors. They are mostly benign but may also be malignant. This group of tumors includes adult and juvenile granulosa cell tumors, Sertoli-Leydig cell tumors, fibromas, thecomas, and sclerosing stromal tumors of the ovary. These tumors are usually not graded except for Sertoli-Leydig cell tumors.

All adult granulosa cell tumors are potentially malignant. Certain microscopic subtypes portend a more aggressive tumors growth. For example, adult granulosa cell tumors that are classified as diffuse (sarcomatoid) have a more aggressive behavior than microfollicular, macrofollicular, insular, or trabecular granulosa cell tumors. Juvenile granulosa cell tumors, if removed in stage I, have an excellent prognosis, but larger and more advanced tumors may progress and have a less favorable outcome. Microscopic grading has no clinical utility in either adult or juvenile granulose cell tumors, but larger tumors.

Ovarian thecomas and fibromas are generally benign tumors. Fibrosarcoma, the malignant equivalent of fibroma, has all the features of malignancy and can be readily distinguished from the benign stromal tumors.

10.13.1 Sertoli-Leydig Cell Tumor

Sertoli-Leydig cell tumors account for less than 1 % of all ovarian tumors. These tumors occur in several microscopic forms that predict their clinical behavior (Prat 2004). Thus, the variants and/or grades of Sertoli-Leydig cell tumors are as follows:

- *Well-differentiated Sertoli-Leydig cell tumor.* This tumor consists of Sertoli cells arranged into tubules, surrounded by fibrous stroma and solid nests of Leydig cells.
- *Sertoli-Leydig cell tumors of intermediate differentiation.* This tumor contains large nests of polygonal Leydig surrounded by immature Sertoli cells. These two components may be focally intermixed, and the Sertoli cells may even form abortive tubules.
- *Poorly differentiated Sertoli-Leydig cells (sarcomatoid variant).* This tumor is composed predominantly of mitotically active, hyperchromatic, and anaplastic stromal cells and scattered foci of Leydig cells.
- *Retiform Sertoli-Leydig cell tumor.* These tumors resemble rete testis and are composed of inter-anastomosing clefts lined by cuboidal cells that often project into the lumen in form of papillae.
- *Sertoli-Leydig cell tumors with heterologous elements.* In about 20 % of cases, Sertoli-Leydig cell tumors contain heterologous, epithelial, or mesenchymal elements.

Most Sertoli-Leydig cell tumors are benign. Poorly differentiated tumors, which account for 10 % of all tumors in this group, are malignant. Adverse prognosis is also heralded by the presence of heterologous stromal elements (e.g., rhabdomyosarcoma cells).

Books and Monographs

Prat J (2004) Pathology of the ovary. Saunders, Philadelphia
Robboy SJ, Mutter GL, Prat J, Bentley RC, Russell P, Anderson MC (eds) (2009) Pathology of the female reproductive tract, 2nd edn. Churchill Livingstone, London
Tavassoli F, Devilee P (eds) (2003) World Health Organization classification of tumours. Pathology and genetics of tumours of the breast and female genital organs, IARC Press, Lyon

Articles

1. Hart WR (2001) Vulvar intraepithelial neoplasia: historical aspects and current status. Int J Gynecol Pathol 20:16–30

2. Lerma E, Matias-Guiu X, Lee SJ, Prat J (1999) Squamous cell carcinoma of the vulva: study of ploidy, HPV, p53, and pRb. Int J Gynecol Pathol 18:191–197

3. Santos M, Montagut C, Mellado B et al (2004) Immunohistochemical staining for p16 and p53 in premalignant and malignant epithelial lesions of the vulva. Int J Gynecol Pathol 23:206–214

4. Cannistra SA, Niloff JM (1996) Cancer of the uterine cervix. N Engl J Med 334:1030–1038

5. Giannoudis A, Herrington CS (2001) Human papillomavirus variants and squamous neoplasia of the cervix. J Pathol 193:295–302

6. Llewellyn H (2000) Observer variation, dysplasia grading, and HPV typing: a review. Am J Clin Pathol 114(Suppl):S21–S35

7. Gray LJ, Herrington CS (2004) Molecular markers for the prediction of progression of CIN lesions. Int J Gynecol Pathol 23:95–96

8. Zaino RJ (2000) Glandular lesions of the uterine cervix. Mod Pathol 13:261–274

9. Young RH, Clement PB (2002) Endocervical adenocarcinoma and its variants: their morphology and differential diagnosis. Histopathology 41:185–207

10. Wheeler DT, Kurman RJ (2005) The relationship of glands to thick wall blood vessels as a marker of invasion in endocervical adenocarcinoma. Int J Gynecol Pathol 24:125–130

11. Catasus L, Gallardo A, Prat J (2009) Molecular genetics of endometrial carcinoma. Diagn Histopathol 15:554–563

12. Prat J (2004) Prognostic parameters of endometrial carcinoma. Hum Pathol 35:649–662

13. Report M (2009) The new FIGO staging system for cancers of the vulva, cervix, endometrium and sarcomas. Gynecol Oncol 115:325–328

14. Clement PB, Young RH (2002) Endometrioid carcinoma of the uterine corpus: a review of its pathology with emphasis on recent advances and problematic aspects. Adv Anat Pathol 9:145–184

15. Bell SW, Kempson RL, Hendrickson MR (1994) Problematic uterine smooth muscle neoplasms. A clinicopathologic study of 213 cases. Am J Surg Pathol 18:535–558

16. D'Angelo E, Prat J (2010) Uterine sarcomas. A review. Gynecol Oncol 116:131–139

17. Downes KA, Hart WR (1997) Bizarre leiomyomas of the uterus: a comprehensive pathologic study of 24 cases with long term follow-up. Am J Surg Pathol 21:1261–1270

18. Alvarado-Cabrero I, Young RH, Vamvakas EC, Scully RE (1999) Carcinoma of the fallopian tube: a clinicopathological study of 105 cases with observations on staging and prognostic factors. Gynecol Oncol 72:367–379

19. Prat J (2012) Ovarian carcinomas: five distinct diseases with different origins, genetic alterations, and clinicopathological features. Virchows Arch 460:237–249

20. Ayhan A, Kurman RJ, Yemelyanova A et al (2009) Defining the cut-point between low- and high-grade ovarian serous carcinomas: a clinicopathologic and molecular genetic analysis. Am J Surg Pathol 33:1220–1224

21. Lee KR, Scully RE (2000) Mucinous tumors of the ovary—a clinicopathologic study of 196 borderline tumors (of intestinal type) and carcinomas, including an evaluation of 11 cases with "pseudomyxoma peritonei". Am J Surg Pathol 24:1447–1464

22. Rodriguez IM, Prat J (2002) Mucinous tumors of the ovary: a clinicopathologic analysis of 75 borderline tumors (of intestinal type) and carcinomas. Am J Surg Pathol 26:139–152

23. Provenza C, Young RH, Prat J (2008) Anaplastic carcinoma in mucinous ovarian tumors: a clinicopathologic study of 34 cases emphasizing the crucial impact of stage on prognosis, their histologic spectrum, and overlap with sarcoma-like mural nodules. Am J Surg Pathol 32:383–389

24. Norris HJ, Zirkin HJ, Benson WL (1976) Immature (malignant) teratoma of the ovary: a clinical and pathologic study of 58 cases. Cancer 37:2359–2372

Tumors of the Breast

11

Fang Fan

11.1 Introduction

Breast carcinoma is the most common malignant tumor in women in North America and Europe. Invasive mammary carcinoma and ductal carcinoma *in situ* should be graded routinely in surgically removed or biopsied tissue samples. The grading of these tumors has considerable clinical significance.

11.2 Ductal Carcinoma In Situ

Ductal carcinoma in situ (DCIS) is considered a precursor of invasive carcinoma. Grading of DCIS is meaningful in predicting recurrence and guiding management. While there is no universally agreed-upon grading system for ductal carcinoma in situ, current practice is to grade DCIS on the basis of nuclear characteristics alone or in combination with necrosis. The architectural histopathologic features are not taken into account for grading of DCIS.

The grading system published in the most recent World Health Organization (WHO) monograph is a three-tiered system based on nuclear grade alone [1]. It incorporates the basic tenets of the so-called Van Nuys grading scheme [2] and

the approach outlined by Scott et al. [3], thus representing the most recent refinement of the original classification published by Lagios et al. in 1989 [4]. It divides DCIS into DCIS of low nuclear grade, DCIS of intermediate nuclear grade, and DCIS of high nuclear grade (Table 11.1). College of American Pathologists (CAP), in an effort to standardize all pathology reports, also recommends specifying in the pathology report the nuclear grade and indicating the presence or absence of necrosis, instead of combining both features for an overall histologic grade [5].

- *Nuclear grade* (Table 11.1) is mainly based on the size of the nuclei, distribution of chromatin, and the presence or absence of nucleoli. Nuclear pleomorphism, nuclear orientation, and mitoses are the additional features that are used in the grading as well.
- *Necrosis* is either present or absent. If present, it typically involves the centrally located cells inside the ducts. Necrotic cells undergo karyorrhexis or pyknosis. These signs of cell death are associated with a loss of nuclear details, clumping of chromatin, and fragmentation of nuclei. The presence of necrosis is associated with the mammographic finding of calcifications because necrosis tends to calcify. CAP recommends [5] reporting the presence of necrosis as central ("comedo") or focal (punctate) (Fig. 11.4):
  - *Central or "comedo" necrosis* – The central portion of an involved duct is filled with a solid expansive area of necrosis that is visible under low power view.

F. Fan, M.D., Ph.D.
Department of Pathology,
The University of Kansas School of Medicine,
Kansas City, KS, USA
e-mail: ffan@kumc.edu

I. Damjanov, F. Fan (eds.), *Cancer Grading Manual*,
DOI 10.1007/978-3-642-34516-6_11, © Springer-Verlag Berlin Heidelberg 2013

Table 11.1 Nuclear grade of ductal carcinoma in situ

Grade	Nuclear features
1.	The nuclei are small, round, and uniform. The nuclei of tumor cell are of the size as the red blood cell or slightly larger. Their diameter does not exceed by more than 1.5 times the diameter of normal red blood cells ($1.5\times$ RBC). The nuclei contain uniformly dispersed chromatin, and the nucleoli are not apparent. Mitoses are rare. The cells are polarized around small lumens or rosette-like structures (Fig. 11.1)
2.	Tumor cell nuclei are enlarged, and their diameter is equivalent to 1.5–2 times the size of red blood cells ($1.5\times$ to $2\times$ RBC). The chromatin is coarse, but the nucleoli are infrequently seen. There are sparse mitoses. Cell polarization around luminal spaces is present (Fig. 11.2)
3.	Tumor cell nuclei have diameters greater than 2.5 red blood cells ($\times2.5$ RBC). The nuclei are vesicular with clumped chromatin and irregular nuclear membrane. There are one or more prominent nucleoli. Mitotic figures may be frequent, but their presence is not required for grading. Cells are not polarized around luminal spaces (Fig. 11.3)

Adapted from Schnitt et al. [1] and College of American Pathologists protocol [5]

- *Focal or punctate* – The necrotic foci are small and may only be single-cell necrosis. It is not easily detected under low magnification.
- Necrosis must be distinguished from inspissated eosinophilic secretions, hemorrhage, foam cells, or debris without karyorrhexis of tumor cells.

11.2.1 Ancillary Methods

Ancillary methods may be used but are not essential for grading of DCIS. They may be useful under certain circumstances to support the diagnosis and exclude other possibilities as follows:

- Immunohistochemical stains for myoepithelial cells, including smooth muscle actin, calponin, and collagen IV, can be helpful in cases when invasion is suspected [6].
- Immunohistochemical stains for E-cadherin and antibody 34βE12 to high-molecular-weight keratin can be helpful in differentiating low-grade solid type DCIS (E-cadherin positive, 34βE12 negative) from lobular neoplasia (E-cadherin negative, 34βE12 positive) [7].
- Immunohistochemical staining for estrogen receptor (ER), progesterone receptor, and HER2 expression may be performed on DCIS for clinical purposes, not for diagnosis or grading. As for invasive carcinomas, these markers identify different molecular types of DCIS including "ER positive," "HER2 posi-

tive," and "triple negative" [8, 9]. The usefulness of this information with regard to prognosis or benefit from treatment is still under investigation [10]. Of note, the majority of DCIS cases (75–80 %) are ER positive.

11.2.2 Comments

1. When more than one grade of DCIS is present, it should be noted in the diagnosis.
2. The architectural pattern of ductal carcinoma in situ (comedo, cribriform, solid, papillary, and micropapillary) should be included in the pathology report because certain patterns carry independent prognostic significance [11]. DCIS of comedo type is associated with high risk of local recurrence and progression to invasive cancer. Micropapillary DCIS may be associated with more extensive disease in multiple quadrants.
3. The status of resection margins and the extent (size) of DCIS are the other two important prognostic factors in the local control of DCIS and should be documented in the pathology report [1].
4. There is no consensus about the grading of uncommon types of DCIS, such as apocrine, clear cell, spindle cell, signet ring, and neuroendocrine types.
5. One must document the presence of microcalcifications and correlate the microscopic findings with mammographic films and/or specimen imaging data.

Fig. 11.1   DCIS of low nuclear grade, cribriform architecture. (**a**) The ducts are distended by a monotonous population of cells with small round to oval nuclei. No central necrosis is present. (**b**) The cells have small nuclei (1–1.5 red blood cells), dispersed chromatin, and inapparent nucleoli (nuclear grade 1)

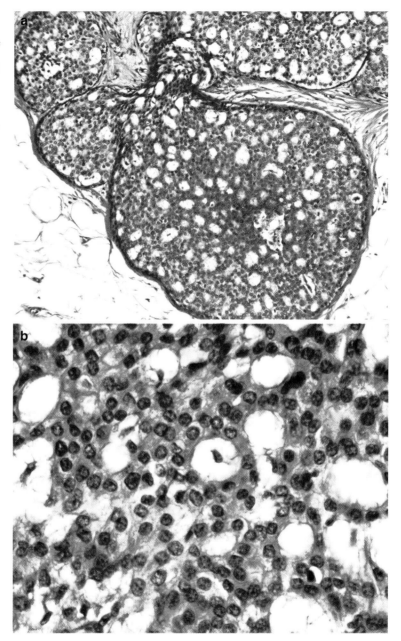

11.3   Lobular Carcinoma In Situ

Tavassoli has proposed a three-level scheme for stratifying lobular intraepithelial neoplasia (LIN 1, LIN 2, and LIN 3) [12]. However, this approach has not been currently endorsed by the experts serving on the WHO panel on breast diseases [13]. Lobular neoplasia is divided into atypical lobular hyperplasia and lobular carcinoma in situ based on the extent of involvement of individual terminal ductal-lobular unit. There is no need for grading lobular carcinoma in situ.

Fig. 11.2 DCIS of intermediate nuclear grade, cribriform architecture. (**a**) The overall pattern is similar to low-grade lesions. There is a central area of necrosis. (**b**) The nuclei are moderately enlarged (1.5–2 red blood cells) with coarse chromatin and occasional prominent nucleoli (nuclear grade 2)

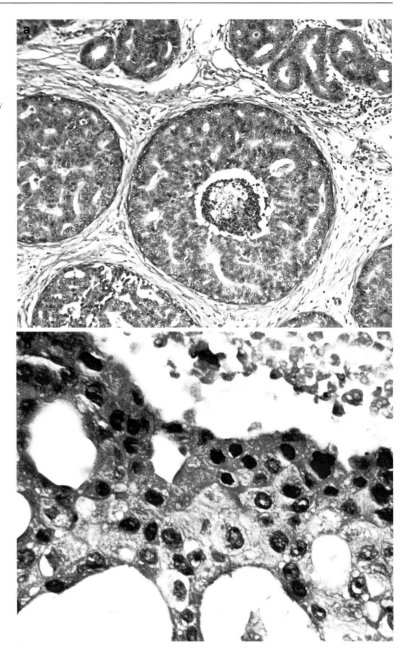

11.4 Invasive Mammary Carcinoma

The relationship between breast cancer morphology or histology and survival was documented in 1920s and 1930s. Greenhough and his colleagues were the first to propose the idea of histologic grading in 1925. These investigators reviewed 73 cases of radical mastectomy specimens and assessed eight morphological factors, including the degree of gland formation; the presence of secretory vacuoles, cell size, and nuclear size; the variation in the size of cells and nuclei; the degree of nuclear hyperchromatism; and the number of mitoses. Tumors were assigned a grade in a three-tier grading system based on the overall evaluation of the above eight features. A clear association between tumor grade and 5-year "cure" was demonstrated. It is fair

Fig. 11.3 DCIS of high nuclear grade, comedo type. (**a**) Extensive central necrosis is surrounded by a rim of highly anaplastic tumor cells. (**b**) The tumor cells have high-grade nuclei (greater than 2.5 red blood cells in diameter) with marked pleomorphism, prominent nucleoli, and mitotic figures (nuclear grade 3)

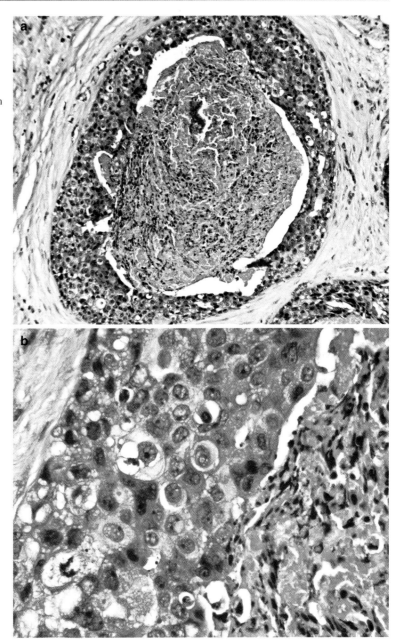

to say that all the current breast grading studies stem from this seminal work.

Patley and Scarff [14] followed Greenhough's method and developed their own grading systems, emphasizing on the amount of tubule formation, variation in nuclear size, and hyperchromatism. They also found associations between grade and survival. However, the idea of breast grading did not gain much popularity among clinicians and pathologists at that time, in part, due to the complexity and subjectivity of the grading system and partly due to the limitation of treatment options corresponding to different grades of the tumor.

In 1950, Bloom (ironically, a radiotherapist) reviewed all literature on breast cancer grading and decided to follow the Patey and Scarff method. He divided tumors into low-, moderate-,

Table 11.2 Histologic grade of invasive breast carcinoma

Features			Score 1	Score 2	Score 3
Formation of tubular and glandular structures			Tubules or glands formed in >75 % of the tumor	Tubules or glands formed in 10–75 % of the tumor	Few if any tubules formed, tubules account for <10 % of the tumor
Nuclear pleomorphism			Tumor nuclei are small, regular, and uniform	Tumor nuclei are moderately increased in size and show variability	Tumor nuclei show marked variation
Mitotic rate (per 10 high-power fields)	Field diameter (mm)	Area (mm^2)			
	0.44	0.152	0–5	6–10	>11
	0.59	0.273	0–9	10–19	>20
	0.63	0.312	0–11	12–22	>23

Adapted from Ellis et al. [17]

Final grade (combining values of the above three features) is calculated as follows:

Grade 1 – Well-differentiated carcinoma. 3–5 points (Fig. 11.4)

Grade 2 – Moderately differentiated carcinoma. 6–7 points (Fig. 11.5)

Grade 3 – Poorly differentiated carcinoma. 8–9 points (Fig. 11.6)

Fig. 11.4 Invasive well-differentiated ductal carcinoma. (**a**) The majority of tumor forms well-recognized tubules/glands (tubule formation >75 %, score 1). (**b**) Tumor nuclei are small and uniform with minimal pleomorphism (nuclear grade 1). Mitosis is rare (score 1). The final histological grade is 3 out of a total score of 9, indicating a grade I (well differentiated) breast carcinoma

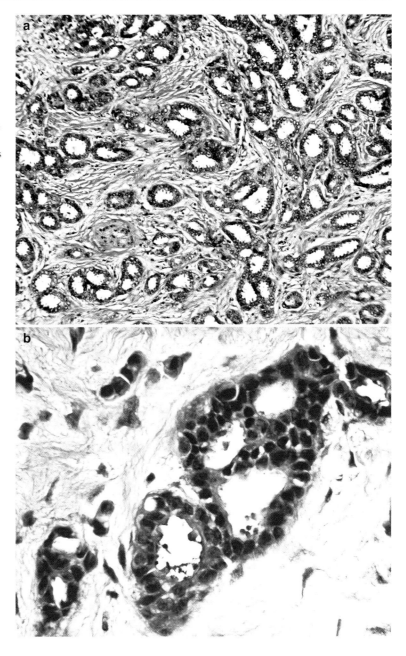

or high-grade malignancy according to the following three factors: (1) the degree of tubule formation; (2) regularity in the size, shape, and staining character of the nuclei; and (3) nuclei hyperchromasia and mitotic activity. He found a clear correlation between tumor grading and 5- and 10-year survival. Following that, in 1957, Bloom and Richardson (a surgical research fellow at that time) first proposed a numerical scoring system to facilitate the grading effort [15]. Each of the above three features was examined and given a score of 1, 2, or 3, with a total possible score of 3–9 points. Then the final grade was arbitrarily assigned as grade I if the score was 3–5, II if the score was 6–7, and III if the score was 8–9. This method was subsequently recommended by the experts of WHO in 1968 as the preferred grading system for breast cancer.

Fig. 11.5 Invasive moderately differentiated ductal carcinoma. (**a**) Tumor cells grow in solid cords and nests with occasional recognizable tubules/glands (tubule formation <10 %, score 3). (**b**) Tumor nuclei are moderately increased in size with mild pleomorphism (nuclear grade 2). Rare mitoses are seen (2/10 high-power field, 0.59 field diameter, score 1). The final histological grade is 6 out of a total score of 9, indicating a grade II (moderately differentiated) breast carcinoma

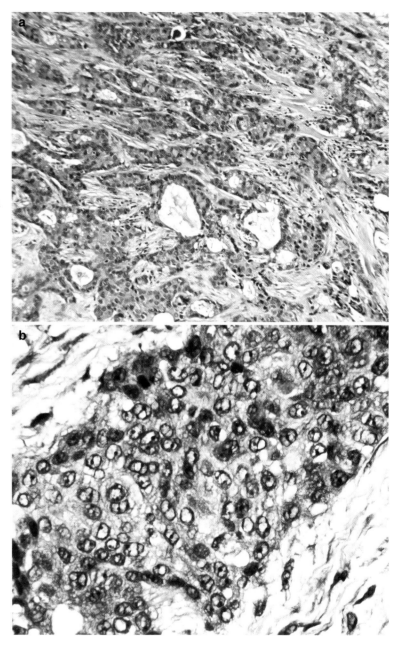

In the mean time, Black and colleagues concluded that only nuclear morphology is the most significant prognostic factor. His nuclear grade evaluation was based on the regularity of the nuclear outline, delicacy of chromatin and nucleoli, and presence and numbers of mitotic figures. However, his five-grade grading system was in reverse numerical order to common practice in that, grades 0 and 1 representing most poorly dif-

ferentiated nuclei. In 1980, Fisher and coworkers modified Black's nuclear grading system by reducing it to a three-grade system and reversing its numerical order to be consistent with other grading scheme. He then combined nuclear grade and tubule formation in evaluating histologic grade of a tumor.

In the early 1990s, Elston and Ellis [16] reexamined the grading system and modified it by

Fig. 11.6 Invasive poorly differentiated ductal carcinoma. (**a**) There is no evidence of glandular formation (tubule formation <10 %, score 3). (**b**) Tumor cells are large with marked pleomorphism (nuclear grade 3). Numerous mitosis is seen with some atypical forms (more than 20 per 10 high-power field, 0.59 field diameter, score 3). The final histological grade is 9 out of a total score of 9, indicating a grade III (poorly differentiated) breast carcinoma

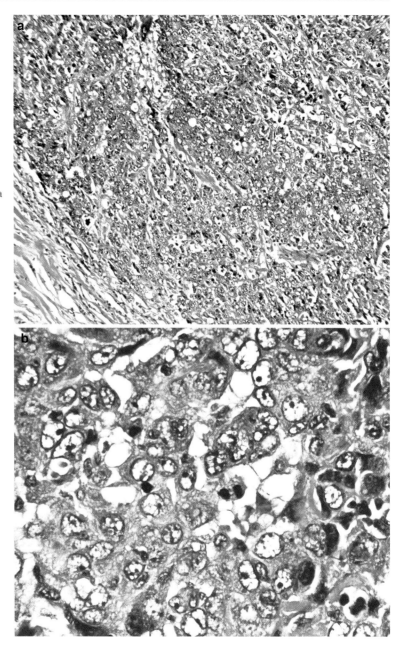

combining the Bloom and Richardson's approach with Black's approach. Most importantly, Elston and Ellis [16] deleted the term "nuclear hyperchromasia," used previously in the Bloom and Richardson's system, and also introduced an objective and numerical method for assessing the mitotic count. They also clearly defined the criteria for other two features, i.e., tubule formation and nuclear pleomorphism. This system, also referred to as Nottingham modification of the Bloom-Richardson system or Elston and Ellis' modification of the Scarff-Bloom-Richardson method, soon gained popularity and currently is used worldwide. It has proven to hold up as a statistically significant clinical prognostic factor. The panel of experts of the WHO has endorsed it, recommending its usage in the pathology reports of all invasive breast cancers.

This semi-quantitative histologic grading system includes three components: evaluation of the extent of the formation of tubules and glands, estimation of the degree of nuclear pleomorphism, and counting of mitoses (Table 11.2).

11.4.1 Ancillary Methods

Ancillary methods are not essential for grading of breast carcinoma but may be used for special purposes as follows:
- Immunohistochemical stains for epithelial and myoepithelial markers can be helpful in cases when invasion is questionable.
- Immunohistochemical stains for E-cadherin can be helpful in differentiating invasive ductal carcinoma (E-cadherin positive) from invasive lobular carcinoma (E-cadherin negative).
- Immunohistochemical staining for estrogen receptor, progesterone receptor, and HER2 expression has prognostic and therapeutic values and should be performed in all invasive carcinoma cases. Although these markers are not used in grading, almost all well-differentiated and most moderately differentiated carcinomas are positive for estrogen receptor and progesterone receptor. Approximately 75–85 % of invasive carcinomas are positive for estrogen receptor, and 15–20 % of invasive carcinomas are positive for HER2 overexpression.
- It has been suggested to use Ki-67 as an objective substitute for mitotic counts in the grading system [18–20].
- Measurement of the degree of genomic instability in breast carcinomas may improve the grading at the genetic level [21].

11.4.2 Comments

1. Nuclear grade is an independent prognostic marker in addition to the histologic grade and should be mentioned separately in the pathology report.

2. Mitotic figures should be counted in ten consecutive high-power fields in the most mitotically active area of the tumor. The size of high-power field must be determined for each microscope with the score categories assigned appropriately [17]. Only clearly identifiable and unequivocal mitoses are counted. Apoptotic nuclei, especially those undergoing karyorrhexis, should not be confused with mitotic figures.
3. All invasive carcinomas, including invasive ductal carcinoma, invasive lobular carcinoma, and special types (medullary carcinoma, tubular carcinoma, mucinous carcinoma, etc.), are graded using this grading system.
4. Molecular studies have shown that the low-grade and high-grade tumors are different diseases with distinct molecular pathways [22, 23].

11.5 Phyllodes Tumors

Phyllodes tumors are biphasic tumors characterized by leaflike structures lined by double-layered epithelial component surrounded by overgrowing hypercellular stroma. Depending on the cellularity and atypia of the stromal component, phyllodes tumors may have features of benign tumors and resemble fibroadenomas or be malignant and share features with breast sarcomas.

Grading of phyllodes tumors is described in detail in the WHO monograph [24]. On the basis of stromal cellularity, cellular pleomorphism, mitotic activity, the appearance of margins, and stromal distribution, the phyllodes tumors are divided into three groups and labeled as benign, borderline, and malignant:
- *Benign phyllodes tumor.* These tumors show modest stromal cellularity, mild cellular pleomorphism, no or only few mitosis (<5 per 10 HPF), and have well-circumscribed pushing margins. The stromal distribution in these tumors is uniform (Fig. 11.7a).
- *Borderline phyllodes tumor.* These tumors show modest stromal cellularity, moderate cellular pleomorphism, and moderate mitotic activity (5–9/10 HPF) and have partially

Fig. 11.7 Phyllodes tumor. (**a**) Benign phyllodes tumor. There is a leaflike structure lined by benign epithelium with underlying cellular stroma. The stroma is composed of uniform spindle cells with only rare mitoses. (**b**) Malignant phyllodes tumor. The stroma is frankly sarcomatous and contains numerous mitotic figures

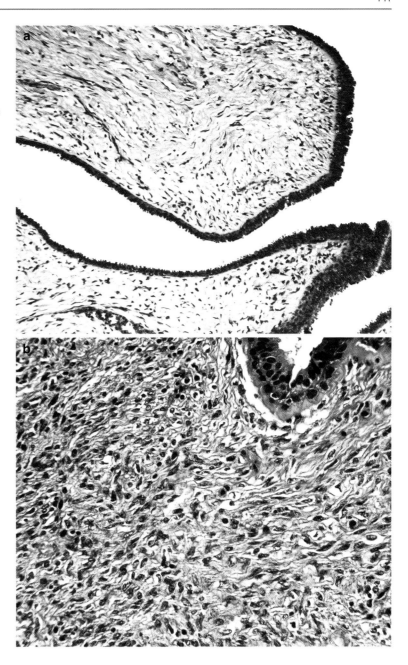

infiltrative margins. There is stromal overgrowth, but it is typically uneven.

- *Malignant phyllodes tumor.* These tumors show marked stromal cellularity, marked cellular pleomorphism, and numerous mitoses (≥ 10/10HPF) and have widely invasive margins. Invariably they show marked stromal overgrowth (Fig. 11.7b).

11.5.1 Ancillary Methods

Ancillary methods are not required for grading of phyllodes tumors. Immunohistochemical stains for several biomarkers, such as MIB-1 (Ki-67), p53, and VEGF, correlate with the tumor grade and may be valuable prognostic factors in malignant phyllodes tumor [25–27].

11.5.2 Comments

1. The term "cystosarcoma phyllodes" is inappropriate and should be abandoned because most of these tumors follow a benign course, and thus the term sarcoma is misleading.
2. Sampling of one block for every 1 cm of maximal tumor dimension is necessary for an accurate grading of phyllodes tumor due to the presence of structural variability in these tumors.
3. Tumors should be graded according to the areas of highest cellularity and atypia.
4. Stromal overgrowth is defined as absence of epithelial elements in at least one low-power field (40×) [28].
5. It has been suggested that the mitotic count be related to the field diameter instead of high-power fields because the size of high-power fields varies among microscopes [29].
6. In malignant phyllodes tumors, the epithelial component may only be identified after examining multiple sections due to overgrowth of the sarcomatous component.
7. The sarcomatous component in malignant phyllodes tumor is usually fibrosarcoma. However, heterologous differentiation including liposarcoma, osteosarcoma, chondrosarcoma, or rhabdomyosarcoma may occur, and such changes should be documented in the diagnostic report.

Books and Monographs

Elston CW, Ellis IO (eds) (1998) Systemic pathology: the breast, vol 13, 3rd edn. Churchill Livingstone, Edinburgh

Lakhani SR, Ellis IO, Schnitt SJ et al (eds) (2012) World Health Organization classification of tumours: pathology of the breast. IARC, Lyon

Tavassoli FA (ed) (1999) Pathology of the breast. Appleton-Lange, Stamford

Articles

1. Schnitt SJ, Allred C, Britton P et al (2012) Ductal carcinoma in situ. In: Lakhani SR, Ellis IO, Schnitt SJ et al (eds) World Health Organization classification of tumours: pathology of the breast. IARC, Lyon, pp 90–94
2. Silverstein MJ, Lagios MD, Craig PH (1996) A prognostic index for ductal carcinoma in situ of the breast. Cancer 77:2267–2274
3. Scott MA, Lagios MD, Axelsson K, Schnitt SJ et al (1997) Ductal carcinoma in situ of the breast: reproducibility of histologic subtype analysis. Hum Pathol 28:967–973
4. Lagios MD, Margolin FR, Westdahl PR et al (1989) Mammographically detected duct carcinoma in-situ: frequency of local recurrence following tylectomy and prognostic effect of nuclear grade on local recurrence. Cancer 63:618–624
5. College of American Pathologists. Protocol for the examination of specimens from patients with ductal carcinoma in situ (DCIS) of the breast. Available at: http://www.cap.org. Accessed on 2 Aug 2012
6. Yaziji H, Gown AM, Sneige N (2000) Detection of stromal invasion in breast cancer: the myoepithelial markers. Adv Anat Pathol 7:100–109
7. Bratthauer GL, Moinfar F, Stamatakos MD et al (2002) Combined E-cadherin and high molecular weight cytokeratin immunoprofile differentiates lobular, ductal and hybrid mammary intraepithelial neoplasm. Hum Pathol 33:620–627
8. Bradley GG, Schnitt SJ, Collins LC (2006) Ductal carcinoma in situ with basal-like phenotype: a possible precursor to invasive basal-like breast cancer. Mod Pathol 19:617–621
9. Steinman S, Wang J, Bourne P et al (2007) Expression of cytokeratin markers, ER-alpha, PR, Her-2/neu, and EGFR in pure ductal carcinoma in situ (DCIS) and DCIS with co-existing invasive ductal carcinoma (IDC) of the breast. Ann Clin Lab Sci 37:127–134
10. Harris L, Fritsche H, Mennel R et al (2007) American Society of Clinical Oncology 2007 update of recommendations for the use of tumor markers in breast cancer. J Clin Oncol 25:5287–5312
11. Bellamy CO (1993) Noninvasive ductal carcinoma of the breast: the relevance of histologic categorization. Hum Pathol 24:16–22
12. Tavassoli FA (1999) Lobular neoplasia. In: Tavassoli FA (ed) Pathology of the breast. Appleton-Lange, Stamford, pp 373–397
13. Lakhani SR, Schnitt SJ, O'Malley F et al (2012) Lobular neoplasia. In: World Health Organization classification of tumours: pathology of the breast. IARC, Lyon, pp 78–80
14. Patey DH, Scarff RW (1928) The position of histology in the prognosis of carcinoma of the breast. Lancet 1:801–804
15. Bloom HJG, Richardson WW (1957) Histologic grading and prognosis in breast cancer: a study of 1709 cases of which 359 have been followed for 15 years. Br J Cancer 2:353–377
16. Elston CW, Ellis IO (1998) Assessment of histological grade. In: Elston CW, Ellis IO (eds) Systemic

pathology: the breast, vol 13, 3rd edn. Churchill Livingstone, Edinburgh, pp 365–384

17. Ellis IO, Simpson JF, Reis-Filho JS, Decker T (2012) Invasive breast carcinoma: introduction and general features – grading. In: Lakhani SR, Ellis IO, Schnitt SJ et al (eds) World Health Organization classification of tumours: pathology of the breast. IARC, Lyon, pp 19–20

18. Trihia H, Murray S, Price K et al (2003) Ki-67 expression in breast carcinoma: its association with grading systems, clinical parameters, and other prognostic factors—a surrogate marker? Cancer 97:1321–1331

19. Tawfik O, Kimler BF, Davis M et al (2007) Grading invasive ductal carcinoma of the breast: advantage of using automated proliferation index instead of mitotic count. Virchows Arch 450:627–636

20. Meyer JS, Alvarez C, Milikowski C et al (2005) Breast carcinoma malignancy grading by Bloom-Richardson system vs proliferation index: reproducibility of grade and advantages of proliferation index. Mod Pathol 18:1067–1078

21. Kronenwett U, Huwendiek S, Ostring C et al (2004) Improved grading of breast adenocarcinomas based on genomic instability. Cancer Res 64:904–909

22. Roylance R, Gorman P, Harris W et al (1999) Comparative genomic hybridization of breast tumors stratified by histologic grade reveals new insights into the biological progression of breast cancer. Cancer Res 59:1433–1436

23. Sotiriou C, Wirapati P, Loi S et al (2006) Gene expression profiling in breast cancer: understanding the molecular basis of histologic grade to improve prognosis. J Natl Cancer Inst 98:262–272

24. Tan PH, Tse G, Lee A et al (2012) Fibroepithelial tumors. In: Lakhani SR, Ellis IO, Schnitt SJ et al (eds) World Health Organization classification of tumours: pathology of the breast. IARC, Lyon, pp 145–146

25. Niezabitowski A, Lackowska B, Rys J et al (2001) Prognostic evaluation of proliferative activity and DNA content in the phyllodes tumor of the breast: immunohistochemical and flow cytometric study of 118 cases. Breast Cancer Res Treat 65:77–85

26. Tan PH, Jayabaskar T, Yip G et al (2005) p53 and c-kit (CD117) protein expression as prognostic indicators in breast phyllodes tumors: a tissue microarray study. Mod Pathol 18:1527–1534

27. Tse GM, Lui PC, Lee CS et al (2004) Stromal expression of vascular endothelial growth factor correlates with tumor grade and microvessel density in mammary phyllodes tumors: a multicenter study of 185 cases. Hum Pathol 35:1053–1057

28. Ward RM, Evans HL (1986) Cystosarcoma phyllodes. A clinicopathologic study of 26 cases. Cancer 58:2282–2289

29. Moffat CJ, Pinder SE, Dixon AR et al (1995) Phyllodes tumors of the breast: a clinicopathological review of thirty-two cases. Histopathology 27:205–218

Lymphoid and Hematopoietic Systems

12

Lawrence M. Weiss and Karen L. Chang

12.1 Introduction

Grading of tumors plays a less significant role in the hematopoietic and lymphoid systems than perhaps any other organ system. While grading was once an integral part of the classification of the non-Hodgkin's lymphomas, it is now considered more relevant to give a precise classification, thereby imparting the information that the clinician requires for prognostication and treatment planning. Nonetheless, there are selected neoplasms in which grading plays an accepted and sometimes important role. In the future, however, ancillary methods such as immunohistochemistry, flow cytometry, and cytogenetics, already of great importance, as well as gene profiling, will likely play an even increasingly critical role in determining prognosis and response to therapy in lymphoid and hematopoietic neoplasms.

12.2 Follicular Lymphoma

Grading of follicular lymphoma has been accepted as having clinical relevance for many years [1–4]. However, the optimal method of grading and the specific clinical implications have yet to be determined. The 2001 World Health Organization (WHO) Classification of Tumours of Haematopoietic and Lymphoid Tissues proposed a specific methodology that, while not validated, provided a standardized methodology (Jaffe et al. 2001). Guidelines for how to apply the grading system were updated in the most recent WHO classification (Swerdlow et al. 2008), which has been used in clinical practice and correlated with the pathophysiology and cell biology of this form of lymphoma [5, 6].

12.2.1 Grading System

According to the 2001 WHO classification, follicular lymphoma is graded by counting the number of centroblasts in ten neoplastic follicles, expressed per 40× high-power microscopic field (hpf), based on a hpf of 0.159 mm^2 (Jaffe et al. 2001). Centroblasts (also called large noncleaved cells) are large lymphoid cells with round to oval and occasionally indented nuclei, a vesicular chromatin pattern, one to three nucleoli usually situated at or near the nuclear membrane, and a narrow rim of cytoplasm. Centroblasts must be distinguished from large centrocytes (large cleaved cells), which also have large nuclei, but a

L.M. Weiss, M.D. (✉)
Department of Pathology,
Clarient Pathologist Services, Inc.,
Aliso Viejo, CA, USA
e-mail: weiss11111@gmail.com

K.L. Chang, M.D.
Department of Pathology,
Kaiser Permanente Southern California,
Los Angeles, CA, USA

I. Damjanov, F. Fan (eds.), *Cancer Grading Manual*,
DOI 10.1007/978-3-642-34516-6_12, © Springer-Verlag Berlin Heidelberg 2013

Fig. 12.1 Follicular lymphoma, grade 1. There is a great predominance of small cleaved lymphoid cells, with only a few centroblasts

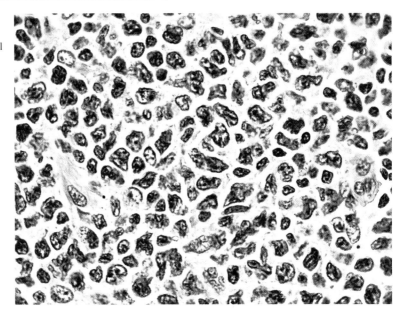

Fig. 12.2 Follicular lymphoma, grade 2. There are scattered centroblasts among the small cleaved lymphoid cells

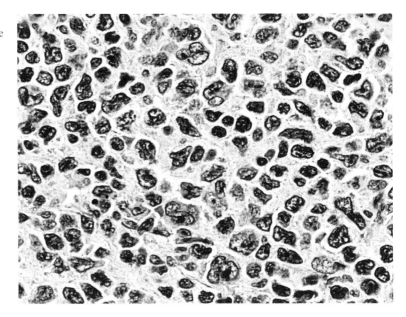

more angulated and elongated nucleus and a more condensed chromatin pattern, with inconspicuous nucleoli, as well as follicular dendritic cells, which are often multinucleate and possess a finer chromatin pattern, nucleoli which tend to be more centrally placed, and a finer nuclear membrane.

The criteria for grade recommended by the WHO are as follows:

Grade 1: 0–5 centroblasts/hpf (Fig. 12.1)
Grade 2: 6–15 centroblasts/hpf (Fig. 12.2)

Grade 3: >15 centroblasts/hpf
(a) Centrocytes still present (Fig. 12.3)
(b) Solid sheets of centroblasts (Fig. 12.4)
The 0.159-mm^2 field is derived from a microscope with a 40× objective and an 18-mm field of view ocular. Appropriate adjustments must be made when using other magnification objectives or different-sized ocular fields. Each high-power field should be counted within a different follicle, without selecting the follicles.

Fig. 12.3 Follicular lymphoma, grade 3a. Although scattered small cleaved lymphoid cells are still present, there is a predominance of centroblasts

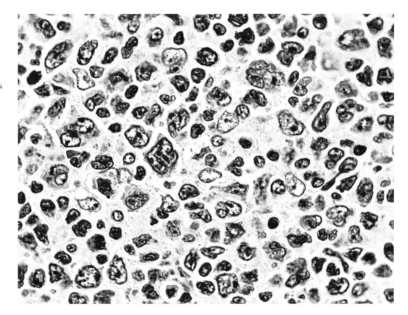

Fig. 12.4 Follicular lymphoma, grade 3b. Virtually all the cells in this neoplastic follicle are centroblasts, without small cleaved lymphoid cells

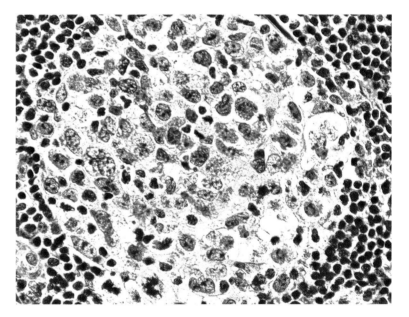

If discrete areas of grade 3 follicular lymphoma are present in a case that is otherwise of lower grade, a second grade is given, with the approximate amount of each grade reported as a percentage.

Diffuse variants of follicular lymphoma are graded 1 and 2, based on the identical criteria given above. There is no grade 3 diffuse variant of follicular lymphoma, as this is regarded as diffuse large B-cell lymphoma.

12.2.2 Comments

Grades 1 and 2 follicular lymphoma are traditionally regarded as indolent or low-grade follicular lymphoma, while grade 3 follicular lymphoma has been shown to behave in a more aggressive fashion and is usually regarded as intermediate grade. Since there are no convincing studies showing a significant difference in survival between grades 1 and 2, but many studies showing substantial interobserver disagreement, the 2008 update to the WHO classification recommended that grades 1 and 2 be combined into a "low-grade" category (Swerdlow et al. 2008).

The cytologic subtypes of grade 3 follicular lymphoma have not been shown to predict survival. Cytogenetic and other studies have suggested that a significant subset of cases of grade 3B follicular lymphoma may be more closely related to diffuse large B-cell lymphomas of germinal center origin rather than other cases of follicular lymphoma [7–11]. This data is consistent with other studies showing that at least some cases of grade 3 follicular lymphoma have the potential for cure with aggressive therapy. However, at least one study found that grade 3B cases have a gene expression profile closer to other cases of follicular lymphoma than diffuse large B-cell lymphoma [12]. The 2008 WHO classification recommends that one attempt to distinguish grade 3A from 3B cases (Swerdlow et al. 2008).

The presence of diffuse areas may have an adverse impact on survival, particularly in grade 3 neoplasms [11]. Transformation (progression to a large B-cell lymphoma) may occur in up to one-third of patients and usually is an ominous finding.

There has been a proposal for a revision of the follicular lymphoma international prognostic index, based on a variety of clinical factors [13]. As yet, there is no comparison between this index and histologic grading in providing prognostic information for the individual patient.

12.3 Mantle Cell Lymphoma

While there is no formal grading system, cases of mantle cell lymphoma can be divided into classic and blastic (blastoid) types (Jaffe et al. 2002). Cases of classic mantle cell lymphoma have a median survival of about 4–5 years, with the majority not curable. In most studies blastic mantle cell lymphoma has a poor prognosis, with a median survival usually less than 2 years.

12.3.1 Grading System

Classical mantle cell lymphoma is composed of a relatively monotonous population of small- to medium-sized lymphoid cells, in either a diffuse, vaguely nodular, or mantle zone distribution. The lymphoid cells have irregular nuclear outlines, a relatively mature lymphoid chromatin pattern with inapparent or inconspicuous nucleoli, and an inapparent rim of cytoplasm (Fig. 12.5). The mitotic rate usually averages about 20 per 10 hpf. Rare variants may show features mimicking the cells of chronic lymphocytic leukemia/small lymphocytic lymphoma or a marginal zone B-cell lymphoma.

There are two main types of blastic mantle cell lymphoma. In the more frequent type, termed by some classic or lymphoblastoid, the cells have a close morphologic resemblance to the cells of precursor lymphoblastic leukemia/lymphoma, with a very fine chromatin pattern, inapparent or inconspicuous nucleoli, and an inapparent rim of cytoplasm (Fig. 12.6). The mitotic rate is greater than 30 per 10 hpf and usually averages 50 per 10 hpf. In the second type, termed by some pleomorphic or large cell, the cells are usually more heterogeneous, with a spectrum from cell resembling those found in typical cases of mantle cell lymphoma to larger cells with larger cleaved to oval nuclei, clearly discernible nucleoli, and a rim of pale cytoplasm (Fig. 12.7). Other cases feature the presence of large blast-like cells and may be virtually indistinguishable from some cases of diffuse large B-cell lymphoma. Thus, the grading of mantle cell lymphoma is given below:

Mantle cell lymphoma
- Typical
- Blastic
  - Classic/lymphoblastoid
  - Pleomorphic/large cell

12.3.2 Ancillary Methods

Cyclin D1 immunohistochemical staining, while not absolutely sensitive or specific, is most useful in confirming the diagnosis of mantle cell

Fig. 12.5 Mantle cell
lymphoma, typical type.
There is a relatively
homogeneous population of
small lymphoid cells with a
relatively mature chromatin
pattern but definite
abnormalities of the nuclear
membrane

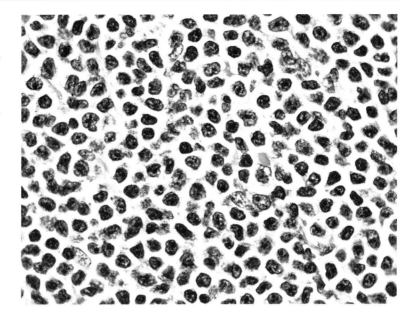

Fig. 12.6 Mantle cell
lymphoma, classical blastic
type. The cells are very
uniform and have a blastic
chromatin pattern, mimicking
a lymphoblastic neoplasm

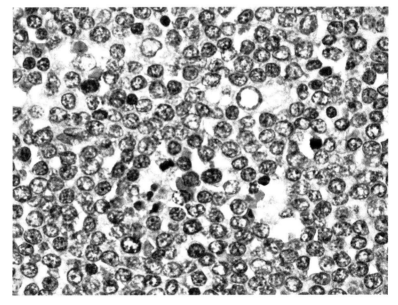

lymphoma. Demonstration of evidence of a
t(11;14) by molecular studies may also be useful.
P27 staining may be useful in the distinction
between typical and blastic variants of mantle cell
lymphoma, as it is usually negative in typical mantle cell lymphoma and positive in blastic mantle
cell lymphoma [14]. Blastic variants of mantle cell
lymphoma also tend to have frequent bcl-1 rearrangements at the major translocation cluster
region, tetraploid chromosome clones, and
increased incidence of p53 mutations and overexpression [15, 16]. Gene array studies have shown
that blastic cases have a lower expression of cas-
pase 7, but an increased expression of TOP1 and
CDK4 as compared to other cases of mantle cell
lymphoma [17].

Fig. 12.7 Mantle cell lymphoma, pleomorphic blastic type. The lymphoid cells are of the size of a large cell lymphoma, but have a fine chromatin pattern

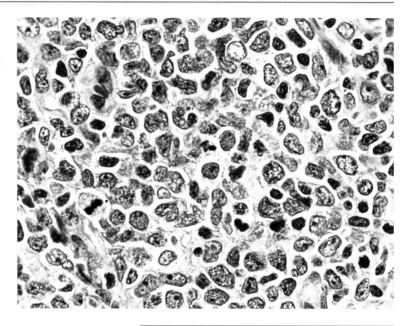

12.3.3 New Developments

Gene expression microarray studies have provided a precise measurement of tumor cell proliferation, provided by the expression of proliferation signature genes, identifying patient subsets that differed by more than 5 years in median survival [18].

12.3.4 Comments

1. When considering a diagnosis of blastic mantle cell lymphoma, it is important to rule out a lymphoblastic malignancy; cyclin D1 and terminal deoxyribonucleotide transferase (TdT) stains are very useful, and the former is highly specific for mantle cell lymphoma, while the latter is highly specific for lymphoblastic malignancies.
2. The large cell variant of mantle cell lymphoma may be easily mistaken for a large B-cell lymphoma. Cyclin D1 staining should be performed in any diffuse large B-cell lymphoma with unusually "cleaved" appearing nuclei or with a relatively evenly dispersed chromatin pattern.
3. Approximately 10–15 % of cases of mantle cell lymphoma will be of the blastic subtype.

12.4 Classical Hodgkin Lymphoma, Nodular Sclerosis Type

Hodgkin lymphoma is currently divided into nodular lymphocyte predominant and classical types (Jaffe et al. 2002). Classical Hodgkin lymphoma, which represents greater than 95 % of cases, is subdivided into nodular sclerosis, mixed cellularity, lymphocyte rich, and lymphocyte depleted forms. With modern therapy, there are no significant differences in prognosis between the different subtypes. The nodular sclerosis subtype represents approximately two-thirds of all cases of classical Hodgkin lymphoma. Therefore, there has been some interest in trying to establish a grading system that can distinguish prognostically significant subgroups within this large group of patients. The most successful grading system has been that proposed by the British National Lymphoma Investigation.

12.4.1 Grading System

The British National Lymphoma Investigation grading of nodular sclerosis classical Hodgkin lymphoma is as follows [19–22]:

Grade 1: All cases not meeting the criteria for grade 2 (Fig. 12.8).

Fig. 12.8 Classical Hodgkin lymphoma, nodular sclerosis, type 1. Note the scattered lacunar Hodgkin cells, which do not form sheets

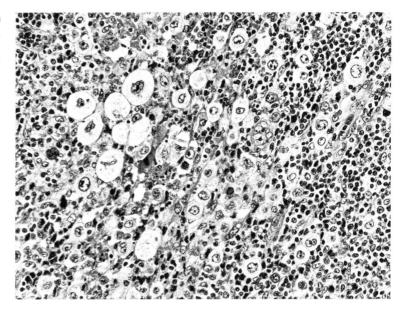

Fig. 12.9 Classical Hodgkin lymphoma, nodular sclerosis, type 2. There is a focus of necrosis, surrounded by sheets of lacunar Hodgkin cells

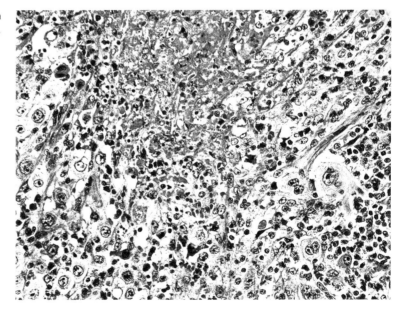

Grade 2:

1. More than 25 % of the cellular nodules show reticular or pleomorphic lymphocyte depletion (Fig. 12.9); or
2. More than 80 % of the cellular nodules show the fibrohistiocytic variant of lymphocyte depletion; or
3. More than 25 % of the nodules contain numerous bizarre and highly anaplastic-appearing Hodgkin's cells without depletion of lymphocytes (sheets of cells filling a 40× hpf).

12.4.2 Comments

1. Grade 2 nodular sclerosis is somewhat similar to what has been termed nodular sclerosis with lymphocyte depletion in some studies [21] and

overlaps with what has been termed the syncytial variant of nodular sclerosis in other studies [23].

2. This system is somewhat hard to learn, although some studies have shown good reproducibility.
3. Some studies have shown that the patients classified as grade 2 have a significantly worse prognosis than those patients classified as grade 1, although other studies have not confirmed this finding. In general, large numbers of patients must be studied for an effect on prognosis to be demonstrated.
4. This grading scheme has, in general, not been extensively used in daily practice. The WHO does not require its use for routine clinical purposes.

12.5 Mycosis Fungoides: Lymph Node Involvement

Mycosis fungoides is a distinctive cutaneous T-cell lymphoma. Aside from skin, lymph nodes are the most common site of involvement. Clinical stage represents the single most important prognostic factor, with stage II representing enlargement of lymph nodes, but no involvement histologically, and stage III representing lymph node involvement documented by histology. Unfortunately, it is extremely difficult to establish a histologic diagnosis of mycosis fungoides involving lymph nodes, particularly when enlarged lymph nodes in these patients generally show extensive

dermatopathic changes. As a way of establishing, several groups of investigators have established a histologic grading system for the assessment of lymph nodes in patients with mycosis fungoides, as a way of communicating degree of certainty in the diagnosis.

12.5.1 Grading System

The grading system includes three categories [24, 25]:

Category I: No involvement by mycosis fungoides
- LN-0: Reactive changes are present, but no atypical lymphocytes are evident.
- LN-1: Only a few atypical lymphoid cells are noted in the paracortex (Fig. 12.10).
- LN-2: Atypical lymphocytes occur both singly or in small clusters, generally of fewer than three to six cells in the paracortex (Fig. 12.11).

Category II: Early involvement by mycosis fungoides
- LN-3: Large clusters of atypical lymphocytes, generally in aggregates of 15 or more cells, are interspersed between and tend to separate the paracortical histiocytes, often accompanied by large immunoblastic cells (Fig. 12.12).

Category III: Massive involvement by mycosis fungoides

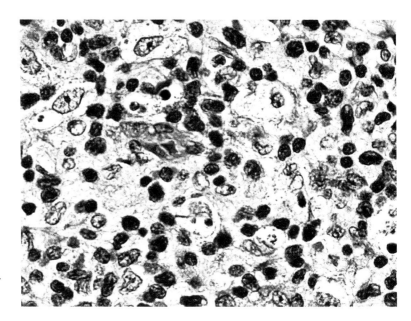

Fig. 12.10 Lymph node involvement by mycosis fungoides, category I, LN-1. Only scattered atypical lymphoid cells are seen

Fig. 12.11 Lymph node involvement by mycosis fungoides, category I, LN-2. Clusters of atypical lymphoid cells are present

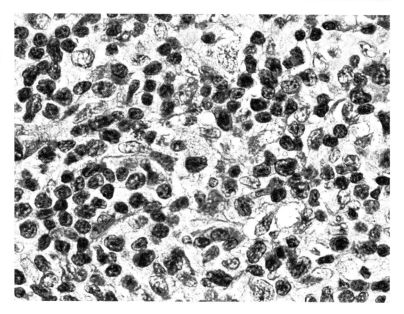

Fig. 12.12 Lymph node involvement by mycosis fungoides, category II, LN-3. Numerous atypical lymphoid cells are seen, but it is still within the context of dermatopathic lymphadenitis

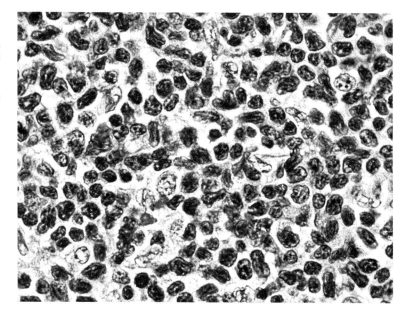

- LN-4: Partial or complete obliteration of architecture by atypical lymphocytes is evident (Fig. 12.13).

12.5.2 Ancillary Techniques

Immunohistochemical studies are of limited utility in establishing a diagnosis of lymph node involvement by mycosis fungoides [26]. Most commonly, aberrant loss of CD7 is seen, but this is not completely specific for mycosis fungoides. Clonal T-cell receptor gene rearrangements can be detected in a subset of cases of Category I, usually those in LN-2, and in the large majority of cases of Category II and III [27–30]. Some studies have suggested that the identification of clonal T-cell populations in Category I lymph nodes may adversely impact prognosis. Therefore, this test is recommended in all Category I lymph nodes, and positive results may be utilized to upstage the patients.

Fig. 12.13 Lymph node involvement by mycosis fungoides, category III, LN-4. There is architectural effacement by sheets of atypical lymphoid cells

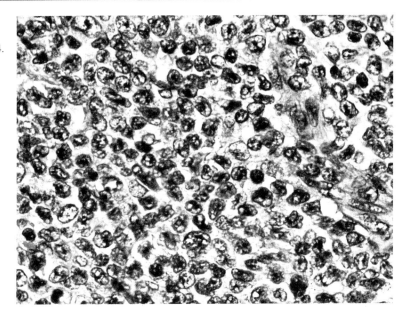

12.5.3 Comments

1. Patients with mycosis fungoides as well as other skin diseases often show changes of extensive dermatopathic lymphadenopathy, due to disruption of the skin barrier. This condition is marked by a proliferation of Langerhans cells and other dendritic cells, histiocytes, and lymphoid cells. Many of these lymphoid cells may have irregular nuclear contours, mimicking the atypical cells seen in mycosis fungoides [31].
2. Scattered immunoblasts may be seen in dermatopathic lymphadenopathy, associated or unassociated with mycosis fungoides. However, when sheets of immunoblasts are present, one must consider the possibility of involvement by mycosis fungoides with large cell transformation, an ominous development associated with a significantly decreased survival period [32].

12.6   Myelodysplastic Syndromes

The myelodysplastic syndromes represent a group of clonal hematopoietic stem cell diseases characterized by abnormal and inefficient hematopoiesis in one or more of the major hematopoietic cell lineages. There may be an increase in the percentage of myeloblasts, but the presence of 20 % or more blasts indicates a diagnosis of acute leukemia rather than a myelodysplastic syndrome. The recent WHO classification recognizes seven specific morphologic subtypes and acknowledges an additional category of myelodysplastic syndrome, unclassified (Jaffe et al. 2002). These subtypes can be stratified into three risk groups based on the duration of survival and incidence of evolution to acute leukemia. Thus, these risk groups represent a kind of grading system.

12.6.1 Grading System

The currently used grading system recognizes three categories: low-grade, intermediate-grade and high-grade lesions.

The group of low-grade forms of myelodysplastic syndromes includes the following:

- *Refractory cytopenia with unilineage dysplasia*: unilineage dysplasia affecting one of the three hematopoietic lines, most commonly the erythroid lineage, with myeloblasts <1 % in the blood and <5 % in the bone marrow (Fig. 12.14)
- *Refractory anemia with ringed sideroblasts (RARS)*: unilineage dysplasia affecting the erythroid lineage, with myeloblasts absent from blood and <5 % in the bone marrow and in which there are >15 % ringed sideroblasts in the bone marrow (Fig. 12.15)

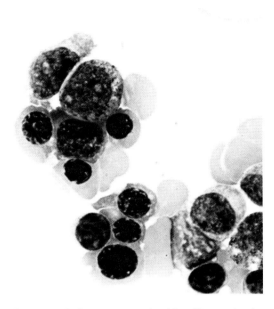

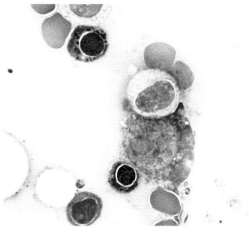

Fig. 12.15 Ringed sideroblasts are characterized by a concentric distribution of fine *blue* granules in this Prussian blue stain

Fig. 12.14 Refractory cytopenia with unilineage dysplasia. The erythroid series shows mild nuclear-to-cytoplasmic dyssynchrony. The myeloid series is *left* shifted but not dysplastic and there are no blasts

Fig. 12.16 Isolated 5q- syndrome. (**a**) The bone marrow core biopsy is slightly hypercellular and shows erythroid and megakaryocytic hyperplasia. (**b**) The megakaryocytes are typically unilobated in this entity

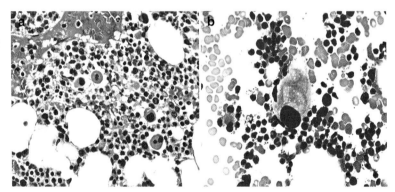

- *Myelodysplastic syndrome associated with isolated del(5q) chromosome abnormality (5q syndrome)*: a clonal proliferation characterized by an isolated del(5q) abnormality in which there are <5 % myeloblasts in the blood and bone marrow (Fig. 12.16a, b)

The group of intermediate-grade forms of myelodysplastic syndromes includes the following:
  - *Refractory cytopenia with multilineage dysplasia (RCMD)*: dysplasia in >10 % of the cells in two or more of the myeloid cell lineages, with <5 % myeloblasts in the marrow, absent Auer rods, and <15 % ringed sideroblasts (Fig. 12.17)
  - *Refractory anemia with multilineage dysplasia and ringed sideroblasts (RCMD-RS)*: same as above with >15 % ringed sideroblasts in the bone marrow.
  - *Refractory anemia with excess blasts-1 (RAEB-1)*: Unilineage or multilineage dysplasia with <5 % blasts in the blood, 5–10 % blasts in the bone marrow, <1 × 10^9/L monocytes, and absent Auer rods (Fig. 12.18).

Fig. 12.17 Refractory cytopenia with multilineage dysplasia. The marrow shows markedly dyssynchronous maturation in the myeloid and erythroid cells but no increase in blasts

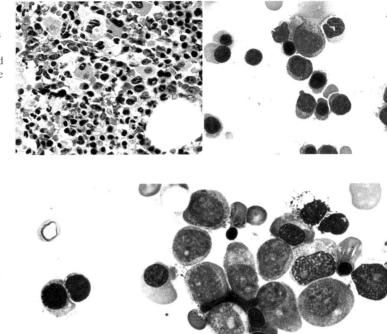

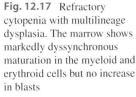

Fig. 12.18 RAEB-1. The dysplastic changes include mild nuclear-to-cytoplasmic dyssynchronous maturation in the erythroid and myeloid series. A rare blast is present

Fig. 12.19 This case of RAEB-2 shows marked dysplasia in the myeloid and erythroid series and an increased number of blasts

The group of high-grade forms of myelodysplastic syndromes includes the following.

- *Refractory anemia with excess blasts-2 (RAEB-2)*: Unilineage or multilineage dysplasia with 5–19 % blasts in the blood, 10–19 % blasts in the bone marrow, and $<1 \times 10^9/L$ monocytes (Fig. 12.19).

12.6.2 Ancillary Studies

Cytogenetics has been shown to be an important prognostic indicator in the myelodysplasia [33]. This variable has been combined with the percentage of blasts and the presence of various cytopenias to derive a scoring system [34]. Favorable prognosis cytogenetics include -Y, del (5q), del (20q), and normal cytogenetics; poor prognosis cytogenetics include complex (>3) or chromosome 7 abnormalities, while intermediate prognosis cytogenetics include all other clonal abnormalities.

12.6.3 Comments

1. In addition to the hematologic findings and cytogenetics, age has been found to be a predictor of survival, with improved survival seen in patients of younger age.
2. The median survival is approximately 5–6 years in RA, RARS, and 5q- syndrome; 3 years in RCMD and RCMD-RS; 1.5 years for RAEB-1; and 1 year for RAEB-2.
3. Although this classification appears to recognize discrete disease entities, this is more appearance than reflecting biologic processes; therefore, some flexibility is required. As the natural history is that of progression, one from a lower grade entity to a higher grade entity as well as from myelodysplastic syndrome to acute leukemia, the disease process should be reevaluated each time additional findings appear.

Books and Monographs

Weiss L (2008) Lymph nodes. Cambridge University Press, Cambridge

Jaffe ES, Harris NL, Stein H, Vardiman JW (2001) World Health Organization classification of tumours. Pathology and genetics – tumours of haematopoietic and lymphoid tissues. IARC Press, Lyon

Swerdlow SH, Campo E, Harris NL et al (2008) World Health Organization classification of tumours. Pathology and genetics – tumours of haematopoietic and lymphoid tissues, 4th edn. IARC Press, Lyon

Articles

1. Anon (1982) National Cancer Institute sponsored study of classification of non-Hodgkin's lymphomas: summary and description of a working formulation for clinical usage. The Non-Hodgkin's Lymphoma Pathologic Classification Project. Cancer 49:2112–2135
2. Mann R, Berard C (1983) Criteria for the cytologic subclassification of follicular lymphomas: a proposed alternative method. Hematol Oncol 1:187–192
3. Metter G, Nathwani B, Burke J et al (1985) Morphological subclassification of follicular lymphoma: variability of diagnosis among hematopathologists, a collaborative study between the Repository Center and Pathology Panel for Lymphoma Clinical Studies. J Clin Oncol 3:25–38
4. Nathwani B, Metter G, Miller T et al (1986) What should be the morphologic criteria for the subdivision of follicular lymphomas? Blood 68:837–845
5. Piccaluga PP, Sapienza MR, Agostinelli C (2009) Biology and treatment of follicular lymphoma. Expert Rev Hematol 2:533–547
6. Stvenson FK, Stvenson GT (2012) Follicular lymphoma and the immune system: from pathogenesis to antibody therapy. Blood 119:3659–3667
7. Bosga-Bouwer A, van Imhoff G, Boonstra R et al (2003) Follicular lymphoma grade 3B includes 3 cytogenetically defined subgroups with primary t(14;18), 3q27, or other translocations: t(14;18) and 3q27 are mutually exclusive. Blood 101:1149–1154
8. Ott G, Katzenberger T, Lohr A et al (2002) Cytomorphologic, immunohistochemical, and cytogenetic profiles of follicular lymphoma: 2 types of follicular lymphoma grade 3. Blood 99:3806–3812
9. Bosga-Bouwer AG, van den Berg A, Haralambieva E et al (2006) Molecular, cytogenetic, and immunophenotypic characterization of follicular lymphoma grade 3B; a separate entity or part of the spectrum of diffuse large B-cell lymphoma or follicular lymphoma? Hum Pathol 37:528–533
10. Katzenberger T, Ott G, Klein T et al (2004) Cytogenetic alterations affecting BCL6 are predominantly found in follicular lymphomas grade 3B with a diffuse large B-cell component. Am J Pathol 165:481–490
11. Hans CP, Weisenburger DD, Vose JM et al (2003) A significant diffuse component predicts for inferior survival in grade 3 follicular lymphoma, but cytologic subtypes do not predict survival. Blood 101:2363–2367
12. Piccaluga PP, Califano A, Klein U (2008) Gene expression analysis provides a potential rationale for revising the histological grading of follicular lymphomas. Haematologica 93:1033–1038
13. Federico M, Bellei M, Marcheselli L et al (2009) Follicular lymphoma international prognostic index 2: a new prognostic index for follicular lymphoma developed by the international follicular lymphoma prognostic factor project. J Clin Pathol 27:4555–4562
14. Quintanilla-Martinez L, Thieblemont C, Fend F et al (1998) Mantle cell lymphomas lack expression of p27Kip1, a cyclin-dependent kinase inhibitor. Am J Pathol 153:175–182
15. Ott G, Kalla J, Ott M et al (1997) Blastoid variants of mantle cell lymphoma: frequent bcl-1 rearrangements at the major translocation cluster region and tetraploid chromosome clones. Blood 89:1421–1429
16. Zoldan M, Inghirami G, Masuda Y et al (1996) Large-cell variants of mantle cell lymphoma: cytologic characteristics and p53 anomalies may predict poor outcome. Br J Haematol 93:475–486
17. Martinez N, Camacho R, Algara P et al (2003) The molecular signature of mantle cell lymphoma reveals multiple signals favoring cell survival. Cancer Res 63:8226–8232
18. Rosenwald A, Wright G, Wiestner A et al (2003) The proliferation gene expression signature is a quantitative integrator of oncogenic events that predicts survival in mantle cell lymphoma. Cancer Cell 3:185–197
19. Bennett M, MacLennan K, Easterling M (1983) The prognostic significance of cellular subtypes in nodular sclerosing Hodgkin's disease: an analysis of 271 non-laparotomised cases (BNLI report no. 22). Clin Radiol 34:497–501
20. MacLennan K, Bennett M, Tu A et al (1989) Relationship of histopathologic features to survival and relapse in nodular sclerosing Hodgkin's disease: a study of 1,659 patients. Cancer 64:1686–1693
21. DeVita V, Simon R, Hubbard S et al (1980) Curability of advanced Hodgkin's disease with chemotherapy. Long-term follow-up of MOPP-treated patients at the National Cancer Institute. Ann Intern Med 92:587–595
22. MacLennan K, Bennett M, Vaughan H (1992) Diagnosis and grading of nodular sclerosing Hodgkin's disease: a study of 2190 patients. Int Rev Exp Pathol 33:27–51
23. Strickler J, Michie S, Warnke R et al (1986) The "syncytial variant" of nodular sclerosing Hodgkin's disease. Am J Surg Pathol 10:470–477
24. Scheffer E, Meijer C, van Vloten W (1980) Dermatopathic lymphadenopathy and lymph node involvement in mycosis fungoides. Cancer 45:137–148

25. Colby T, Burke J, Hoppe R (1981) Lymph node biopsy in mycosis fungoides. Cancer 47:351–359

26. Weiss L, Wood G, Warnke R (1985) Immunophenotypic differences between dermatopathic lymphadenopathy and lymph node involvement in mycosis fungoides. Am J Pathol 120:179–185

27. Weiss L, Hu E, Wood G et al (1985) Clonal rearrangements of the T cell receptor gene in mycosis fungoides and dermatopathic lymphadenopathy. N Engl J Med 313:539–544

28. Bakels V, Van Oostveen J, Geerts M et al (1993) Diagnostic and prognostic significance of clonal T-cell receptor beta gene rearrangements in lymph nodes of patients with mycosis fungoides. J Pathol 170:249–255

29. Lynch J, Linoilla I, Sausville E et al (1992) Prognostic implications of evaluation for lymph node involvement by T-cell antigen receptor gene rearrangement in mycosis fungoides. Blood 79:3293–3299

30. Kern D, Kidd P, Moe R et al (1998) Analysis of T-cell receptor gene rearrangement in lymph nodes of patients with mycosis fungoides. Prognostic implications. Arch Dermatol 134:158–164

31. Burke J, Colby T (1981) Dermatopathic lymphadenopathy. Comparison of cases associated and unassociated with mycosis fungoides. Am J Surg Pathol 5:343–352

32. Vergier B, de Muret A, Beylot-Barry M et al (2000) Transformation of mycosis fungoides: clinicopathological and prognostic features of 45 cases. French study group of cutaneous lymphomas. Blood 95:2212–2218

33. Willman C (1998) Molecular genetic features of myelodysplastic syndromes (MDS). Leukemia 12(Suppl):S2–S6

34. Greenberger J, Crocker A, Vawter G et al (1997) International scoring system for evaluating prognosis in myelodysplastic syndromes. Blood 89:2079–2088

Tumors of the Soft Tissue and Bone 13

Zoran Gatalica, John F. Fetsch, Markku Miettinen, and Ivan Damjanov

13.1 Introduction

Tumors of the soft tissues and bones form a het-erogeneous group that includes on one hand com-mon benign neoplasms and, on the other less common, variably malignant neoplasms (sarco-mas). Recent advances in molecular and cell biology have considerably influenced the present clinical approach to these tumors. As the classifications of these tumors and most notably soft tissue sarcomas constantly change and are refined by the addition of new data, the grading of soft tissue and bone sarcomas remains a work in progress [1, 2]. Accordingly we shall present only the most established grading systems used in daily surgical pathology practice.

Z. Gatalica, M.D., D.Sc (✉)
Department of Pathology,
Creighton University School of Medicine,
Omaha, NE, USA

Caris Life Sciences, Phoenix, AZ, USA
e-mail: zgatalica@carisls.com

J.F. Fetsch, M.D.
Soft Tissue Pathology, The Joint Pathology Center,
606 Stephen Sitter Ave., Silver Spring,
20910-1290, MD, USA

M. Miettinen, M.D.
National Cancer Institute, Bethesda, MD, USA
e-mail: markku.miettinen@nih.hhs.gov

I. Damjanov, M.D., Ph.D.
Department of Pathology,
The University of Kansas School of Medicine,
Kansas City, KS, USA
e-mail: idamjano@kumc.edu

13.2 Soft Tissue Sarcomas

Grading of soft tissue sarcomas (STS) had been controversial for years, primarily because of uncertainty of how to uniformly apply the grading principles to the diverse variety of soft tissue neo-plasms and how to weigh the importance of factors such as differentiation level, mitotic rate, and tumor necrosis. The system that was introduced in 1984 by Costa et al. [3], later known as the National Cancer Institute (NCI) system, was widely used in the USA. The grading system proposed by French Federation of Cancer Centers (Federation Nationale des Centres de Lutte Contre le Cancer, FNCLCC) [4, 5] has gained considerable popular-ity in many countries of Europe and according to some accounts is the most widely used system [6]. It is also validated by the largest number of patients studied and its reproducibility tested with a large number of participating pathologists [7].

The prognostic value of the NCI and FNCLCC systems were compared in a series of 410 adult patients with soft tissue sarcomas with follow-up [8]. The prognostic value of both systems was examined using univariate and multivariate (Cox's model) analyses, and special attention was devoted to tumors with discordant grades. In univariate analysis, both the NCI and FNCLCC systems were of prognostic value to predict metastasis development and tumor mortality. In multivariate analysis, high-grade tumors, irre-spective of the system used, size ≥10 cm, and deep location were found to be independent prog-nostic factors for the advent of metastases. Tumor

Table 13.1 Grading systema of the French Federation of Cancer Centers

	Score
Tumor differentiation (according to Table 13.2)	1–3
Well-differentiated tumors	1
Defined histogenetic types	2
Poorly differentiated tumors and undefined histogenetic types	3
Mitotic count	
0–9/10 hpf	1
10–19/10 hpf	2
≥20/10 hpf	3
Tumor necrosis	
None	0
≤50 %	1
>50 %	2
Histologic grade	Sum of the preceding scores
I	2 or 3
II	4 or 5
III	6, 7, or 8

Modified from Guillou et al. [7]

Abbreviations: *hpf* high-power field

[a]This grading system formulates the overall grade based on total points of scores from tumor differentiation, mitotic rate, and tumor necrosis

Table 13.2 Tumor differentiation score (according to the updated version of the French Federation of Cancer Centers grading system)

Differentiation score 1

Well-differentiated sarcoma (fibrosarcoma, liposarcoma, leiomyosarcoma, chondrosarcoma), well-differentiated MPNST[a]

Differentiation score 2

Conventional fibrosarcoma

Myxoid sarcomas (MFH, liposarcoma, chondrosarcoma)

Storiform-pleomorphic MFH

Conventional leiomyosarcoma

Well-differentiated malignant hemangiopericytoma

Conventional angiosarcoma

Conventional MPNST

Differentiation score 3

Poorly differentiated fibrosarcoma

Giant cell and inflammatory MFH

Round cell liposarcoma

Pleomorphic sarcomas (liposarcoma, leiomyosarcoma)

Rhabdomyosarcoma (except spindle cell in children)

Poorly differentiated and epithelioid angiosarcoma

Triton tumor, epithelioid MPNST

Extraskeletal mesenchymal chondrosarcoma

Extraskeletal osteosarcoma

Ewing family tumors

Synovial sarcoma

Clear cell sarcoma

Epithelioid sarcoma

Alveolar soft part sarcoma

Malignant rhabdoid tumor

Conventional malignant hemangiopericytoma

Poorly differentiated MPNST

Undifferentiated sarcoma

Dedifferentiated liposarcoma[b]

Modified from Coindre [5] and Guillou et al. [7]

Abbreviations: *MPNST* malignant peripheral nerve sheath tumor, *MFH* malignant fibrous histiocytoma

[a]See Comment 1 in Sect 13.2.1

[b]Low-grade dedifferentiation in liposarcomas may be seen in minority of cases, but the survival rates do not significantly differ between high- and low-grade dedifferentiation [11]

grade had a higher predictive value than size or depth, and higher prognostic weight was assigned to the FNCLCC grading system in Cox's models. Grade discrepancies were observed in 34.6 % of the cases. An increased number of grade 3 STS, a reduced number of grade 2 STS, and a better correlation with overall and metastasis-free survival within subpopulations with discordant grades were observed in favor of the FNCLCC system.

Many issues remain unresolved in both of these systems [2, 9] and neither FNCLCC nor NCI system has been formally endorsed by either the World Health Organization (WHO) or the Association of Directors of Anatomic and Surgical Pathology (ADASP) [10]. However, the French system which is more precisely defined appears as the more reproducible system for practicing pathologists [2].

French Federation of Cancer Centers (FNCLCC) grading system of soft tissue sarcomas of adults is based on the total score obtained from the summation of points for three factors:

differentiation, mitotic rate, and tumor necrosis (Table 13.1).

Each soft tissue sarcoma type has been assigned 1–3 points for differentiation based on the histologic type and level of differentiation (so-called differentiation score, Table 13.2). The mitotic count per 10 high-power fields is

Fig. 13.1 Myxoid tumors.
(**a**) Low-grade myxosarcoma.
(**b**) High-grade myxosarcoma

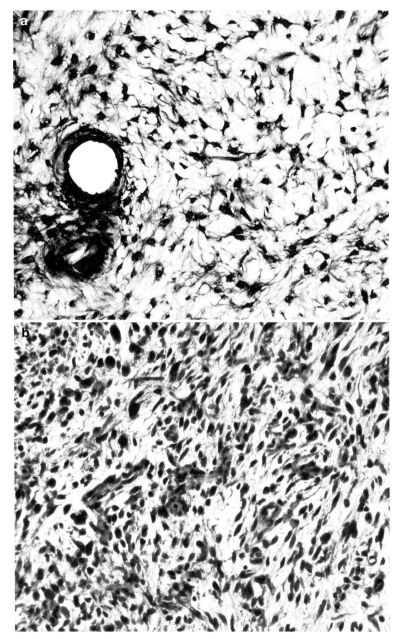

used to assign an additional 1–3 points, and the extent of tumor necrosis (absent, less than half of submitted tumor material or more than half of tumor material) provides for the final 0–2 points. The sum of the all points then determines the tumor grade (2 or 3 points for low grade (grade I), 4 or 5 points for intermediate grade (grade II), and 6 or more points for high grade (grade III)).

Examples of a low-grade and a high-grade myxofibrosarcoma are shown in Fig. 13.1.

The Pediatric Oncology Group grading system for nonrhabdomyosarcomatous soft tissue sarcomas in children [12] addresses issues specific for childhood sarcomas and is given in Table 13.3. It significantly relies on histologic type as the basis for grade, especially for low-grade (grade 1) and high-grade (grade 3) neoplasms.

Table 13.3 The Pediatric Oncology Group grading system for nonrhabdomyosarcomatous soft tissue sarcomas of children

Grade 1

Dermatofibrosarcoma protuberans

Infantile fibrosarcoma, well differentiated (children not over age 4 years)

Infantile hemangiopericytoma, well differentiated

Well-differentiated and myxoid liposarcoma

Well-differentiated MPNST

Extraskeletal myxoid chondrosarcoma

Angiomatoid (malignant) fibrous histiocytoma

Grade 2

Sarcomas not included in grades 1 and 3 with <15 % of necrosis with no more than 5 mitoses/10 hpf

No marked atypia, no markedly high cellularity[a]

Includes noninfantile fibrosarcomas, poorly differentiated infantile fibrosarcomas, leiomyosarcomas, and MPNSTs fitting these criteria

Grade 3

Round cell and pleomorphic liposarcoma

Mesenchymal chondrosarcoma

Extraskeletal osteosarcoma

Malignant triton tumor

Alveolar soft part sarcoma

Sarcomas not included in grade 1 with >15 % of necrosis or with >5 mitoses/10 hpf

Modified from Parham et al. [12]

Abbreviations: *MPNST* malignant peripheral nerve sheath tumor, *MFH* malignant fibrous histiocytoma, *hpf* high-power field

[a]Marked atypia and cellularity may also result in assignment into grade 3

It also incorporates the extent of necrosis and mitotic counts as grading parameters in some (but not all) histologic types as follows:

- *Grade 1 pediatric tumors.* This group is defined by certain histologic types alone, regardless of their cytologic features, amount of necrosis, or mitotic activity.
- *Grade 2 pediatric tumors.* This group is formed for tumors that do not belong to group 1 or group 3 by virtue of histologic diagnosis or the fact that they have <5 mitoses/10 hpf and or <15 % geographic necrosis.
- *Grade 3 pediatric tumors.* This group contains certain tumors known to be clinically aggressive by virtue of histologic diagnosis and non-grade 1 tumors with >4 mitoses/10 high-power fields or >15 % necrosis.

This grading system may result in underestimating the potential of cellular myxoid liposarcoma, which is placed unconditionally in the low-grade group.

13.2.1 Comments

1. Although grading could in principle be applied to any sarcoma type, it has been specifically validated for only the more common tumors, especially spindle cell sarcomas. For malignant peripheral nerve sheath tumors, grading was not found to provide significant prognostic information in the most recent FNCLCC series [5]. However, Wong et al. [13] reported that tumor size, grade, and histologic subtype were independent predictive factors for distant disease control in a series of 134 cases of MPNST.

2. There are no studies to address the grading of rare sarcomas, such as epithelioid sarcoma, clear cell sarcoma, and alveolar soft part sarcoma. However, assuming low mitotic rate and limited if any necrosis, these tumors would generally be assigned an intermediate grade, given their differentiation scores of 3.

3. Limited or inadequate sampling impairs the accuracy of grading and can make it impracticable. Ideal sampling is generally considered to be one histologic section per each centimeter of greatest tumor diameter. Needle biopsies or other small biopsies can only give a minimum grade due to the potentially nonrandom distribution of mitoses, necrosis, and overall differentiation. Because gross sampling of tumors is frequently biased against the inclusion of necrosis, the percentage of necrosis is often underestimated from histologic sections. The most accurate estimate on necrosis would ideally be made based on gross observations, radiologic studies, or by randomized sampling.

4. Counting of mitoses has not been universally standardized, and there is considerable interobserver variability as to what constitutes a mitotic figure. Sometimes karyorrhectic debris and pyknotic or apoptotic nuclei may be

counted. Also, mitotic figures in nonneoplastic components should be excluded. The obtained counts may also depend on microscope field size; the number of counted fields should be adjusted keeping in mind that the field size of 0.174 mm^2 was used to establish the grading system. The level of effort in screening the sections for mitotically most active areas and section thickness may also influence the mitotic counts.

5. Definition of tumor necrosis can be problematic. In the FNCLCC grading system, necrosis related to ulceration, surgery, or hemorrhage has been excluded for consideration.

6. Grading is generally not practicable in post-chemotherapy or post-radiation specimens, as the treatment tends to reduce mitotic counts, increase necrosis, and sometimes seemingly induce differentiation or cause selection for more differentiated components.

7. Different tumor types in the same histologic grade can markedly vary in their metastatic potential. This is perhaps most evident in the low-grade (Grade 1) tumors. For example, well-differentiated lipoma-like liposarcomas have no metastatic potential, whereas even the best-differentiated or least cellular variants of myxoid liposarcoma have significant metastatic potential.

8. Tumor stage is a description of extent of tumor, and it also incorporates grade as one element, as defined in the current TNM and the American Joint Committee for Cancer Staging System for Soft Tissue Sarcomas; the two systems have merged. The other elements of stage are tumor size (whether over 5 cm or not), depth (whether superficial/suprafascial or deep/infrafascial), and localized or disseminated (presence or absence of lymph node and distant metastases).

9. Some histopathologic characteristics other than those used in the grading may be prognostically important. Status of surgical margins is one of the strongest predictors of local recurrence in soft tissue tumors, and the presence of vascular invasion whether intratumoral or extratumoral has been shown as an adverse prognostic factor for some tumor types [14].

10. Numerous studies have suggested cell cycle parameters to have prognostic significance [15, 16]. Among these, proliferation index by Ki-67 analogs detecting cells that have entered the cell cycle and immunohistochemically determined p53 (over)expression are reported to have prognostic significance, but there is no data to support the systematic application of these results to the diagnosis and grading of sarcomas, in general.

11. Gene expression cDNA arrays will very likely provide additional parameters of assessing the biologic potential of soft tissue sarcomas, in addition to their contribution toward biologically more accurate tumor classification [17–20]. Many of these parameters could be assessable by tissue immunohistochemistry, as it has been already shown to be feasible for some leiomyosarcomas [21].

12. Gene expression studies, combined with mutation analyses, can also identify potential therapeutic targets in soft tissue sarcomas. Similar treatments will probably become available for other soft tissue sarcomas in the future. The growing availability of new and often tumor-specific treatments emphasizes importance of accurate classification and grading.

13. Separate from grading, a *managerial classification* has been introduced for soft tissue tumors (see Kempson et al. 2001). This divides different tumor types into clinically benign, intermediate, and sarcoma categories. Each category is subdivided into subcategories based on expected frequencies of recurrence or metastasis and generally advisable treatment types.

14. Recently, nomograms which assess multiple clinical and histologic parameters including tumor size, site, depth, histologic type, grade (low vs. high), and patient age have been used to extrapolate prognosis [22].

13.3 Bone Tumors

Bone tumors are a heterogeneous group including neoplasms of bone-forming, cartilaginous, and other mesenchymal cells. There is no unified histologic grading system for bone sarcomas [23], but the overall emphasis is on a multidisciplinary approach involving not only pathologists but also radiologists and orthopedic surgeons and molecular biologists (for discussion, see Fletcher et al. 2002). There are also radiology-based grading systems that principally assess the tumor aggressiveness by cortical destruction and sclerotic versus permeative margins.

Perhaps the best developed grading system for bone sarcomas is the one used by Mayo Clinic [24]. This system has adapted the principles of Broders, who originally described grading for squamous cell carcinoma of lip and subsequently applied it to fibrosarcoma. The elements of grading are as follows:

- Cellularity (the relative ratio of cells to extracellular matrix)
- Nuclear atypia (enlargement, hyperchromasia, and irregularity of nuclear contours)
- Mitotic count
- Presence and extent of tumor necrosis

Representative, well-processed, and sectioned material should be used for grading. Grading should be carefully preceded by histologic diagnosis and assessment whether benign or malignant based on synthesis of histologic, clinical, and radiologic information. Histologic grading can generally be applied to pretreatment material only. The grading applies to osteosarcoma, fibrosarcoma, malignant fibrous histiocytoma, leiomyosarcoma, chondrosarcoma, and hemangioendothelioma/angiosarcoma. According to the Mayo Clinic system, osteosarcoma, fibrosarcoma, and MFH are assigned grades 1–4, and chondrosarcoma and angiosarcoma/hemangioendothelioma are assigned grades 1–3.

For clinical purposes, bone tumors are best classified as low-grade and high-grade sarcomas as follows:

- *Low-grade sarcomas.* These tumors are generally characterized by low level of nuclear atypia, abundant extracellular matrix (e.g., collagen, osteoid, mineralized bone, and cartilaginous matrix), and low to moderate cellularity. Occasional mitoses are found.
- *High-grade sarcomas.* These tumors are cellular and produce variable amounts of abnormal, immature, and disorganized matrix. The neoplastic cell populations are often pleomorphic or anaplastic, and mitotic activity is often brisk. Necroses are prominent.

Microscopic grade is required for the evaluation and staging of bone sarcomas according to the American Joint Committee on Cancer (AJCC), which recognizes five categories as listed in Table 13.4. For sake of expediency the clinical designation should also be included.

Some bone tumor types are assigned grade by histologic type alone, either because there is limited variation within the tumor type or because attempted grading has not yielded prognostically significant information (Table 13.5). Some specific types of osteosarcoma and chondrosarcomas are also by definition classified as low or high grade. Multiple myeloma and lymphomas of the bone are exempted from grading.

Osteosarcoma. On the basis of clinical-pathologic data, osteosarcomas can be divided into three major groups as follows:

- Conventional (central or medullary) osteosarcoma. These tumors occur in several histologic forms including osteoblastic, chondroblastic, fibroblastic, telangiectatic, small cell, giant cell rich, and epithelioid osteosarcomas.
- Intramedullary (central) well-differentiated osteosarcoma.
- Surface (cortical and parosteal) osteosarcoma.

The grade of osteosarcoma is to a large extent determined by subtype (Table 13.6). Most conventional central (medullary) osteosarcomas are high-grade lesions. Low-grade central osteosarcomas occur infrequently. The opposite is true for cortical and parosteal lesions, among which low-grade variants, such as parosteal osteosarcoma, dominate. Periosteal osteosarcoma, a rare subtype that typically features chondroblastic differentiation, often with high-grade features, is exempted from grading; this tumor has a rather favorable prognosis.

Microscopic features of high-grade and low-grade osteosarcomas are illustrated in Figs. 13.2 and 13.3.

Chondrosarcoma. Several systems for grading chondrosarcomas have been proposed, but none of them has been generally accepted (for discussion, see Fletcher et al. 2002). Once the malignant

Table 13.4 Grading according to the AJCC classification of bone tumors

Grade	Microscopic designation	Clinical designation
GX	Grade cannot be assessed	–
G1	Well differentiated	Low-grade tumor
G2	Moderately differentiated	Low-grade tumor
G3	Poorly differentiated	High-grade tumor
G4	Undifferentiated[a]	High-grade tumor

Modified from American Joint Committee on Cancer (2010) AJCC cancer staging handbook, 7th edn. Springer, New York
[a]Ewing sarcoma is always assigned to the G4 group

Table 13.5 Primary bone tumors other than osteo- and chondrosarcoma that are exempted from formal grading but sometimes assigned a definitional grade

Low grade by definition	High grade by definition	Exempted from grading
Adamantinoma	Ewing family of tumors	Myeloma
Chordoma[a]		Lymphoma

[a]Transformation into high-grade tumors can occur, and occasionally some tumors are high grade from inception

Table 13.6 Grading principles for osteosarcoma

Low grade by definition[a]	High grade by definition[a]
Parosteal osteosarcoma[b]	Conventional medullary osteosarcoma
Low-grade central (medullary) osteosarcoma	High-grade surface osteosarcoma
	Telangiectatic osteosarcoma
	Small cell osteosarcoma

[a]Low-grade tumors are divided into grades 1 and 2 and high-grade tumors into grades 3 and 4 subjectively based on cellularity and atypia
[b]High-grade dedifferentiation may occur

nature of the cartilage forming neoplasm is established based on correlation between radiologic, clinical, and histopathologic evidence, grading should be performed based on cellularity, cytologic features of the chondrocytes, and mitotic activity [25–27]. Necrosis can be seen, particularly in high-grade neoplasms. Conventional chondrosarcomas are graded on a scale of 1–3: 60 % are grade 1, 35 % grade 2, and 5 % grade 3. Clear cell chondrosarcoma is low grade and mesenchymal chondrosarcoma is high grade by definition:

- *Grade 1 chondrosarcoma.* These tumors have well-developed chondroid matrix resulting in low cellularity, which is nevertheless higher than that of typical enchondromas (Fig. 13.4a). The chondrocyte nuclei are small, round, and densely staining. Some nuclei may be slightly enlarged and contain nucleoli. Isolated areas with some pleomorphism are not indicative of a higher grade, as long as there is no increased cellularity and mitotic activity. The peripheral margins are irregular and infiltrative rather than round and well circumscribed. Myxoid degeneration of matrix is considered to be helpful in distinguishing low-grade chondrosarcoma from enchondroma [27]. All clear cell chondrosarcomas are considered to be low-grade tumors [28].

- *Grade 2 chondrosarcoma.* These tumors are moderately cellular (Fig. 13.4b). The nuclei are twice the size of normal chondrocytes and there are occasional mitoses (less than 2 per 10 hpf). The nuclei have irregular contours and appear either hyperchromatic or vesicular with clearly visible nucleoli. Binucleate cells are readily found. Cellularity is particularly prominent at the edges of the tumor lobules.

- *Grade 3 chondrosarcomas.* These tumors are hypercellular and show mitotic activity in excess of 2 per 10 hpf (Fig. 13.4c). High cellularity and pleomorphism may obscure the chondroid nature of some of these tumors. The nuclei are hyperchromatic, contain nucleoli, and show prominent pleomorphism. Bizarre multinucleated cells may be present. Mesenchymal chondrosarcoma and dedifferentiated chondrosarcoma are by definition considered to be high-grade tumors and are included in this group.

Other spindle cell sarcomas. Primary osseous fibrosarcomas, malignant fibrous histiocytomas, and leiomyosarcomas may be graded in a manner similar to those already described for their soft tissue counterparts, although 3-tier grading could be modified to a 4-tier system All these tumors are rare, and the microscopic grade does not seem to influence the clinical course of the disease and prognosis of these tumors. Angiosarcoma, whose low-grade variants are often termed as hemangioendotheliomas, has a spectrum for low to high grade. Grading is based on the degree of vasoformation and endothelial cell atypia, with necrosis and the degree of mitotic activity also being factors.

Fig. 13.2 High-grade osteosarcoma. (**a**) The tumor contains scant extracellular matrix. (**b**) The tumor contains well-developed extracellular matrix, but the cells show prominent hyperchromasia and pleomorphism of their nuclei

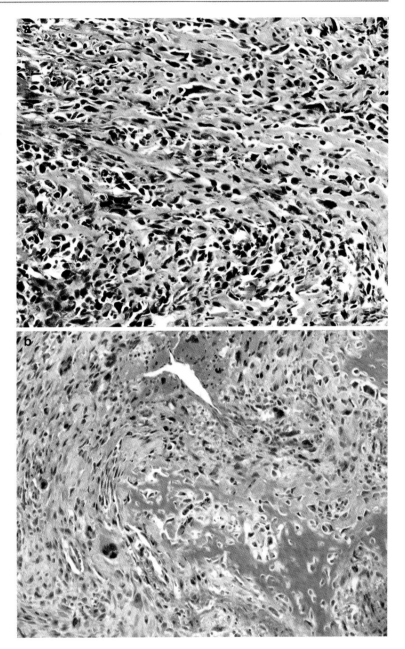

13.3.1 Comments

1. Microscopic examination of osteosarcomas provides limited predictive information about the response of a particular tumor to chemotherapy and radiotherapy. Recently it has been reported that immunohistochemistry with the antibodies to P16 could predict better a favorable response of osteosarcomas to therapy, thus enabling the therapeutic team to distinguish responder (defined as more than 90 % necrosis) from nonresponders [29].

2. Grading of chondrosarcomas is marred by considerable interobserver variability, and new approaches are explored to improve the diagnosis and grading of these tumors [27].

3. The contributions of molecular biology studies to the grading of bone tumors and sarcomas in general are promising but still hard to evaluate objectively [30, 31].

Fig. 13.3 Low-grade parosteal osteosarcoma. The tumor cells are enclosed in a well-developed matrix

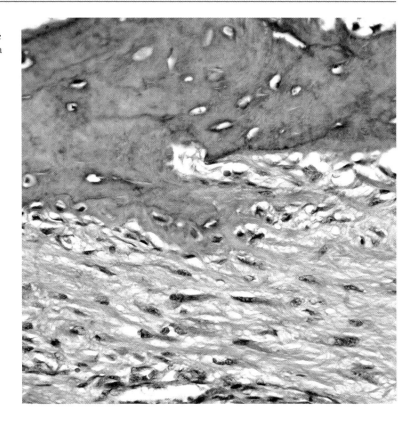

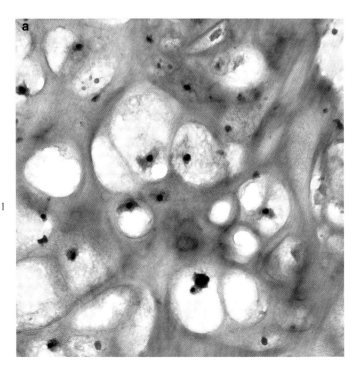

Fig. 13.4 Chondrosarcoma. (**a**) Grade 1 tumor composed of relatively uniform cells with small nuclei. The cells are enclosed by well-developed matrix. (**b**) Grade 2 tumor shows increased cellularity. The tumor cell nuclei are enlarged and show mild to moderate pleomorphism and hyperchromasia. (**c**) Grade 3 tumor. This tumor is composed of spindle-shaped atypical large cells that bear almost no resemblance to cartilage cells

Fig. 13.4 (continued)

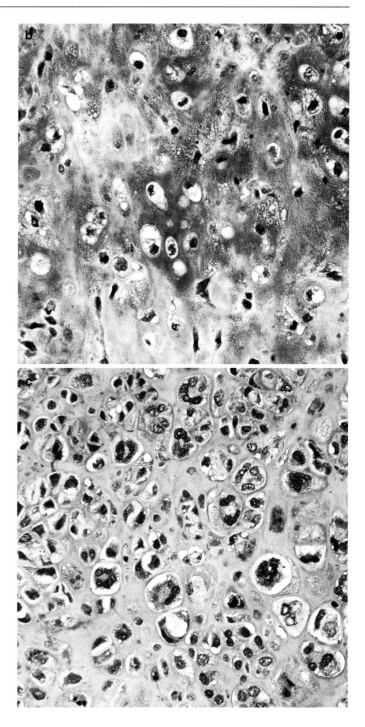

4. Models for treatment and prognosis of sarcomas, like the "Sving" model (acronym for Size, Vascular Invasion, Necrosis, and Growth pattern), have been devised without explicit reference to tumor grading [32]. This multimodality approach appears promising, but the initial data need to be validated. It remains to be determined if the microscopic grading of sarcomas could be used to refine such models.

Books and Monographs

Edge SB, Byrd DR, Compton CC, American Joint Committee on Cancer et al (2010) AJCC cancer staging manual, 7th edn. Springer, New York

Fletcher CDM, Unni KK, Mertens F (eds) (2002) World Health Organization classification of tumours. Pathology and genetics of tumours of soft tissue and bone. IARC Press, Lyon

Miettinen M (2010) Modern soft tissue pathology: tumors and non-neoplastic conditions. Cambridge University Press, Cambridge

Weiss SW, Goldblum JR (2008) Enzinger's and Weiss's soft tissue tumors, 5th edn. Mosby Elsevier, Philadelphia

Articles

1. Fletcher CD (2006) The evolving classification of soft tissue tumours: an update based on the new WHO classification. Histopathology 48:3–12
2. Deyrup AT, Weiss SW (2006) Grading of soft tissue sarcomas: the challenge of providing precise information in an imprecise world. Histopathology 48:42–50
3. Costa J, Wesley RA, Glatstein E, Rosenberg SA (1984) The grading of soft tissue sarcomas. Results of a clinicopathologic correlation in a series of 163 cases. Cancer 53:530–541
4. Trojani M, Contesso G, Coindre JM et al (1984) Soft-tissue sarcomas of adults; study of pathological prognostic variables and definition of a histopathological grading system. Int J Cancer 33:37–42
5. Coindre J-M (2006) Grading of soft tissue sarcoma. Review and update. Arch Pathol Lab Med 130:1448–1453
6. Golouh R, Bracko M (2001) What is the current practice in soft tissue sarcoma grading? Radiol Oncol 35:47–52
7. Coindre JM, Trojani M, Conteso G et al (1986) Reproducibility of a histopathologic grading system for adult soft tissue sarcoma. Cancer 58:306–309
8. Guillou L, Coindre J-M, Bonichon F et al (1997) Comparative study of the National Cancer Institute and French Federation of Cancer Centers Sarcoma Group grading systems in a population of 410 adult patients with soft tissue sarcoma. J Clin Oncol 15:350–362
9. Oliveira AM, Nascimento AG (2001) Grading of soft tissue tumors: principles and problems. Skeletal Radiol 30:543–559
10. Association of Directors of Anatomic and Surgical Pathology (1998) Recommendations for the reporting of soft tissue sarcomas. Mod Pathol 11:1257–1261
11. Henricks WH, Chu YC, Goldblum JR, Weiss SW (1997) Dedifferentiated liposarcoma: a clinicopathological analysis of 155 cases with a proposal for an expanded definition of dedifferentiation. Am J Surg Pathol 21:271–281
12. Parham DM, Webber BL, Jenkins JJ 3rd et al (1995) Nonrhabdomyosarcomatous soft tissue sarcomas of childhood: formulation of a simplified system for grading. Mod Pathol 8:705–710
13. Wong W, Hirose T, Scheithauer BW, Schild SE, Gunderson LL (1998) Malignant peripheral sheath tumor: analysis of treatment outcome. Int J Radiat Oncol Biol Phys 42:351–360
14. Gustafson P, kerman M, Alvergard TA et al (2003) Prognostic information in soft tissue sarcoma using size, vascular invasion and microscopic tumour necrosis – the SIN system. Eur J Cancer 39:1568–1576
15. Hasegawa T, Yamamoto S, Yokoyama R et al (2002) Prognostic significance of grading and staging systems using MIB-1 score in adult patients with soft tissue sarcoma of the extremities and trunk. Cancer 95:843–851
16. Tateishi U, Hasegava T, Beppu Y et al (2003) Prognostic significance of grading (MIB-1 system) in patients with myxoid liposarcoma. J Clin Pathol 56:579–582
17. Nielsen TO, West RB, Linn SC et al (2002) Molecular characterization of soft tissue tumours: a gene expression study. Lancet 239:1301–1307
18. Segal NH, Pavlidis P, Antonescu CR et al (2003) Classification and subtype prediction of adult soft tissue sarcoma by functional genomics. Am J Pathol 163:691–700
19. Antonescu CR (2006) The role of genetic testing in soft tissue sarcoma. Histopathology 48:13–21
20. Taylor BS, Barretina J, Maki RG et al (2011) Advances in sarcoma genomics and new therapeutic targets. Nat Rev Cancer 11:541–557
21. Mills AM, Beck AH, Montgomery KD et al (2011) Expression of subtype-specific group 1 leiomyosarcoma markers in a wide variety of sarcomas by gene expression analysis and immunohistochemistry. Am J Surg Pathol 35:583–589
22. Mariani L, Miceli R, Kattan MW et al (2005) Validation and adaptation of a nomogram for predicting the survival of patients with extremity soft tissue sarcoma using a three-grade system. Cancer 103:402–408
23. Hogendoorn PC, Collin F, Daugaard S, Pathology and Biology Subcommittee of the EORTC Soft Tissue and Bone Sarcoma Group et al (2004) Changing concepts in the pathological basis of soft tissue and bone sarcoma treatment. Eur J Cancer 40:1644–1654
24. Inwards CY, Unni KK (1995) Classification and grading of bone sarcomas. Hematol Oncol Clin North Am 9:545–569
25. Evans HL, Ayala AG, Romsdahl MM (1977) Prognostic factors in chondrosarcoma of bone. A clinicopathologic analysis with emphasis on histologic grading. Cancer 40:818–831
26. Welkerling H, Kratz S, Ewerbeck V, Delling G (2003) A reproducible and simple grading system for classical chondrosarcomas. Analysis of 35 chondrosarcomas and 16 enchondromas with emphasis on recurrence

rate and radiological and clinical data. Virchows Arch 443:725–733

27. Eefting D, Schrage YM, Geirnaerdt MJ et al (2009) Assessment of interobserver variability and histologic parameters to improve reliability in classification and grading of central cartilaginous tumors. Am J Surg Pathol 33:50–57

28. Meijer D, de Jong D, Pansuriya TC et al (2012) Genetic characterization of mesenchymal, clear cell, and dedifferentiated chondrosarcoma. Genes Chromosomes Cancer 51:899–909

29. Borys D, Canter RJ, Hoch B, Martinez SR et al (2012) P16 expression predicts necrotic response among patients with osteosarcoma receiving neoadjuvant chemotherapy. Hum Pathol 43:1948–1954

30. Bovée JV, Hogendoorn PC (2010) Molecular pathology of sarcomas: concepts and clinical implications. Virchows Arch 456:193–199

31. Szuhai K, Cleton-Jansen AM, Hogendoorn PC et al (2012) Molecular pathology and its diagnostic use in bone tumors. Cancer Genet 205:193–204

32. Carneiro A, Bendahl PO, Engellau J et al (2011) A prognostic model for soft tissue sarcoma of the extremities and trunk wall based on size, vascular invasion, necrosis, and growth pattern. Cancer 117:1279–1287

Tumors of the Skin

14

Garth R. Fraga

14.1 Introduction

Skin tumors are the most common neoplasms in humans. Though rarely graded, they are often subtyped. The clinical behavior of some subtypes may vary from that of others, and these differences in outcome and prognosis form the basis for assigning them a pathological grade. I will discuss in this chapter the grading and subtyping of basal cell carcinoma, squamous cell carcinoma, and melanocytic neoplasms.

14.2 Basal Cell Carcinoma

Basal cell carcinoma (BCC) is the most common cutaneous malignant neoplasm in Caucasians. It is considered a malignant neoplasm because it may produce extensive local tissue destruction, but it almost never metastasizes. It has a predilection for the head and neck region of the elderly, but may occur in other sites as well. It is comprised of basaloid cells that demonstrate hair follicle-like differentiation. Though not formally graded, basal cell carcinomas can be subtyped into categories associated with a low and high risk of local recurrence.

G.R. Fraga, M.D.
Department of Pathology,
The University of Kansas School of Medicine,
Kansas City, KS, USA
e-mail: gfraga@kumc.edu

14.2.1 Subtypes of Basal Cell Carcinoma

Numerous subtypes of BCC have been described in the literature. Most cases can be reported as one of five subtypes associated with either a low or high risk of local persistence and tissue destruction. Most basal cell carcinomas are comprised of a mixture of subtypes. Only superficial and nodular subtypes occur as pure populations.

- *Superficial basal cell carcinoma (low risk).* The predominant growth pattern in 28 % of BCC, either as the sole growth pattern or admixed with other growth patterns. Superficial BCC presents as an erythematous patch with a predilection for the trunk and extremities. Biopsies demonstrate small follicle-like buds of basaloid cells arising from the epidermis and limited to the papillary dermis (Fig. 14.1). There are often signs of regression in the papillary dermis between tumor buds consisting of fibrosis, dilated blood vessels, loss of adnexa, and a perivascular infiltrate of lymphocytes and plasma cells [1].
- *Nodular basal cell carcinoma (low risk).* The predominant growth pattern in 60 % of BCC, either as the sole growth pattern or admixed with other growth patterns. Nodular BCC produces raised pearly nodules with a predilection for the head and neck. Histopathology demonstrates expansile round to oval circumscribed nodules of basaloid cells, some discontinuous with the epidermis and associated with epidermal elevation (Fig. 14.2). Cystic,

Fig. 14.1 Superficial basal
cell carcinoma is a flat lesion
comprised of small aggregates
of basaloid cells that bud from
the epidermis and are
separated by intervening
zones of regression comprised
of inflammation and
telangiectasias

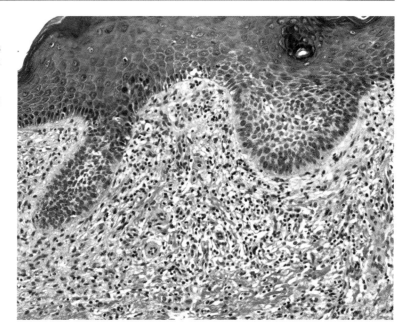

Fig. 14.2 Nodular basal cell
carcinoma is a raised lesion
comprised of nodular dermal
tumor aggregates, some of
which are not contiguous with
the epidermis

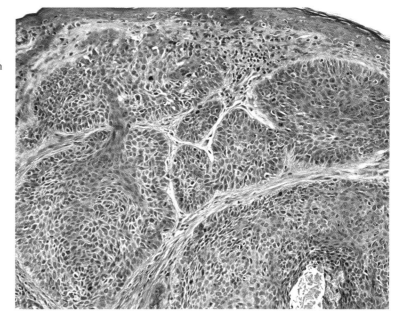

cribriform, or necrotic changes may be present within the tumor cell aggregates, but the periphery of the tumor aggregates is smooth and circumscribed.

- *Infiltrating basal cell carcinoma (high risk).* The predominant growth pattern in 8 % of BCC. Usually it is admixed with a nodular BCC growth pattern. It is characterized by irregular stellate dermal tumor aggregates with spiky contours (Fig. 14.3). Peritumoral mucinous stroma with epithelial-stromal clefting is less common than in superficial or nodular BCC. Some infiltrating BCCs acquire a fibrosing stroma comprised of eosinophilic collagen.

Fig. 14.3 Infiltrating basal
cell carcinoma is comprised of
irregular dermal tumor
aggregates with spiky
contours

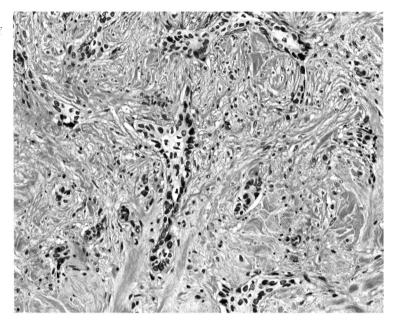

Fig. 14.4 Morpheic/
sclerosing basal cell carcinoma is comprised of widely
infiltrating narrow strands of
basaloid cells, sometimes with
keloidal collagen

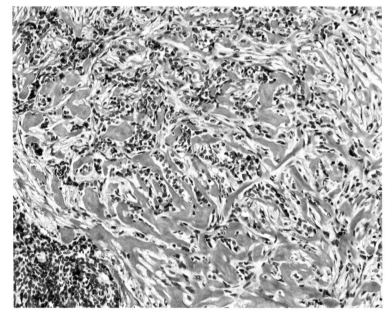

- *Morpheic basal cell carcinoma (high risk).* The
  predominant growth pattern in 2 % of BCC. It
  shares many features of infiltrating BCC, but the
  tumor aggregates are comprised of narrow
  strands ≤2 cells thick (Fig. 14.4). In comparison
  with the infiltrating BCC, it often shows more
  prominent loss of peritumoral mucinous stroma
  or acquisition of an eosinophilic fibrosing
  stroma. Sometimes the peritumoral stroma is
  comprised of thick hyalinized collagen bundles
  similar to those of a keloid; such cases are
  termed "sclerosing basal cell carcinomas."
- *Micronodular basal cell carcinoma (high risk).*
  The predominant growth pattern in 2 % of BCC.

Fig. 14.5 Micronodular basal
cell carcinoma is comprised
of small nodules of tumor
cells that widely infiltrate the
dermis and are not associated
with stromal clefting
or fibromyxoid tumor stroma

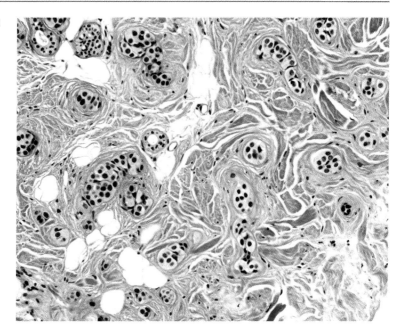

It is defined by small round tumor aggregates <0.15 mm in diameter that widely infiltrate the reticular dermis and are not associated with peritumoral mucinous stroma or epithelial-stromal clefting (Fig. 14.5). There is usually no significant fibro-inflammatory reaction to the infiltrating tumor cells.

14.2.2 Comments

- Signs of tumor regression that are transected in a surgical specimen should be considered evidence of a positive margin.
- Pleomorphic tumor cells, necrosis, and high mitotic index are sometimes seen in basal cell carcinomas, but do not impact prognosis and are not incorporated into tumor grade or subtype.
- The key to accurate diagnosis of micronodular basal cell carcinoma is not only the small widely infiltrative nests of tumor cells but also the absence of a significant stromal reaction to the tumor cells.

14.3   Squamous Cell Carcinoma

Squamous cell carcinoma (SCC) is the second most common malignant cutaneous neoplasm [2–8]. Approximately 2,500 patients in the United

States die annually from metastatic cutaneous SCC. It is an epithelial neoplasm comprised of keratinocytes that recapitulate epidermal differentiation. They are often graded as well, moderately, and poorly differentiated. Poor differentiation is recognized by the American Joint Commission on Cancer (AJCC) as a high-risk feature and incorporated into tumor staging.

- *Well-differentiated SCC.* Sharply demarcated, it is composed of relatively uniform ovoid nests of squamoid cells with abundant dense eosinophilic cytoplasms. Less than 25 % cells are hyperchromic showing a high nuclear-cytoplasmic ratio. Tumor cells form rare keratin pearls comprised of whorls of parakeratin. There is minimal single-cell invasion.
- *Moderately differentiated SCC.* These tumors show greater variation in size and shape of nests. Approximately 25–75 % cells are hyperchromic with high nuclear-cytoplasmic ratios. Nuclear atypia is more pronounced with occasional coarse irregular clumping of nucleoplasm, more striking nuclear hyperchromasia, and more single-cell invasion. Keratin pearls comprised of parakeratin are present, but horn cysts comprised of orthokeratin are absent.
- *Poorly differentiated SCC.* These tumors are comprised of more than 75 % hyperchromic cells showing a high nuclear-cytoplasmic ratio. Poorly differentiated SCC widely

Fig. 14.6 Verrucous squamous cell carcinoma is a large bulky tumor with a papillated surface comprised of aggregates of bland-appearing tumor cells that invade deeply into the skin

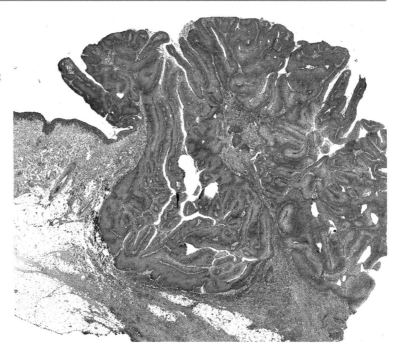

infiltrates the skin with little nesting. There may be extensive single-cell invasion of the underlying dermal connective tissue or deeper soft tissues. Keratinization is often inconspicuous and cytologic atypia is prominent.

14.3.1 Subtypes of Squamous Cell Carcinoma

Squamous cell carcinoma subtypes can be also categorized as low risk (<2 % risk of metastasis) and high risk (>10 % risk of metastasis):

- *Actinic squamous cell carcinoma (low risk).* This by far is the most common form of SCC. It is induced by ultraviolet light and related to sun exposure. Typically, this form of SCC develops from actinic keratosis and has a predilection for the face, dorsal hands, and scalp. They mimic actinic keratoses at the cellular level but demonstrate architectural signs of dermal invasion such as a desmoplastic stromal reaction; undermining growth beneath normal epithelium; jagged, irregular borders; and extension into the reticular dermis (which can be demarcated as the area below the insertion point of the sebaceous gland in a hair follicle). Solar elastosis is always present.

- *Verrucous SCC (low risk).* These tumors are sometimes associated with HPV and have a predilection for anogenital and plantar skin and the oral mucosa. They have a verrucous silhouette and are comprised of bland squamous epithelium invading the underlying dermis/submucosa (Fig. 14.6). This invasion is best demonstrated by comparing the tumor depth to the epithelial-stromal interface in the flanking skin/mucosa.

- *Invasive Bowen disease (high risk).* Bowen disease is an intraepidermal carcinoma comprised of crowded pleomorphic cells with hyperchromatic nuclei forming bizarre mitoses at all levels of the epidermis. Tumor cells are haphazardly arranged, though sparing of a "picket fence" basal cell layer may be seen and is helpful in differentiating Bowen disease from poorly differentiated actinic keratosis. Bowen disease is rarely (<5 %) associated with dermal invasion, which typically presents in form of nests of basaloid cells, often with central comedonecrosis (Fig. 14.7). These nests may exhibit adnexal differentiation. Metastases are found in 13–20 % of patients.

- *SCC arising in damaged skin/Marjolin's ulcer (high risk).* Both exogenous (thermal burn) and endogenous skin injury (discoid lupus erythematosus, lichen sclerosis, stasis ulcer) increases the future risk of SCC in the damaged

Fig. 14.7 Invasive Bowen disease is a high-grade form of squamous cell carcinoma that is comprised of crowded pleomorphic and hyperchromic cells that form invasive tumor aggregates, sometimes with central comedonecrosis and adnexal differentiation

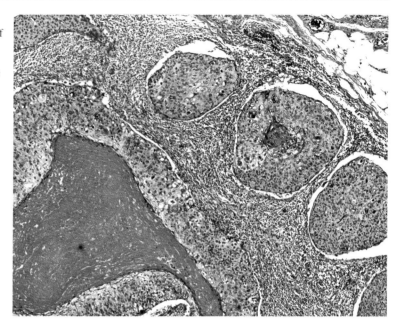

skin. SCC arising in damaged skin is associated with significant risk of lymph node metastases, which are found in 30–50 % of patients. Metastatic SCC is poorly responsive to chemotherapy or radiotherapy.

- *Spindle cell SCC (high risk).* A rare, extremely poorly differentiated sarcomatoid form of SCC that is comprised of elongated spindle cells that widely infiltrate the dermis. There is extensive single-cell invasion with little evidence of squamous differentiation (Fig. 14.8). Spindle cell SCC may mimic melanoma or sarcoma, and the diagnosis often requires immunohistochemical demonstration of high-molecular-weight cytokeratin (e.g., with the antibody to keratin 34β-E12). Antibodies to p63, which is expressed in squamous cell carcinomas but not in sarcomas, are also useful [9].
- *Desmoplastic SCC (high risk).* This rare form of SCC consists of widely infiltrating trabecular cords of tumor cells best seen at the periphery of the tumor, where they are associated with a brisk desmoplastic stromal reaction [8]. Desmoplastic SCC mimics morpheic BCC, from which it differs by showing keratin pearl formation and single-cell keratinization. Epithelial-stromal clefts seen in BCC are not

found in desmoplastic SCC. Lymph node metastases occur in 22 % of patients.
- *Adenosquamous carcinoma (high risk).* This very rare subtype of SCC demonstrates mixed squamous and glandular differentiation (Fig. 14.9). Glandular differentiation can be confirmed with mucicarmine, cytokeratin 7, or CEA. Local recurrence rates between 22 and 26 % are reported, though distant metastases are rare.

14.3.2 Comments

1. Two or more high-risk features upgrade SCC from T1 to T2 in the 2010 AJCC staging classification. High-risk features include poor differentiation, perineural invasion, location on the ear or hair-bearing lip, Breslow thickness >2 mm, and Clark level ≥IV.
2. Though tumor thickness is probably the most important predictor of behavior of cutaneous SCC, it is rarely reported by pathologists. SCC <2 mm in thickness almost never metastasizes, SCC between 2 and 5 mm in thickness gives rise to metastases in 5 % of patients, and SCC >5 mm in thickness produces metastases in 20 % of patients. Pathologists should

Fig. 14.8 Spindle cell
squamous carcinoma may be
morphologically indistin-
guishable from desmoplastic
melanoma and cutaneous
sarcoma; diagnosis depends
upon identifying usual SCC in
a part of the tumor or
demonstrating keratin or p63
expression by
immunohistochemistry

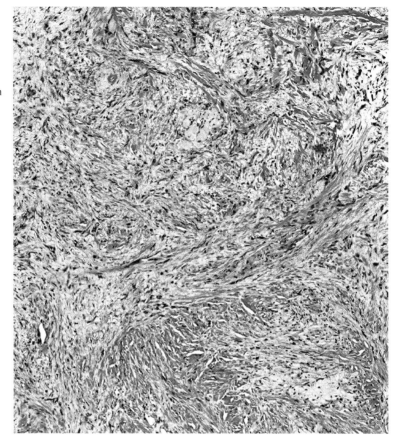

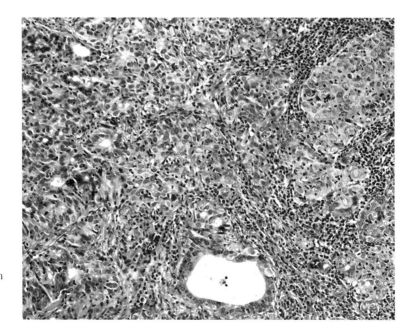

Fig. 14.9 Adenosquamous
carcinoma is a biphasic form
of squamous cell carcinoma
that includes a complement
of gland-forming cells

consider reporting tumor thickness in SCCs, particularly in those with a Breslow thickness >2 mm or subcutaneous invasion.

3. Though commonly considered a variant of SCC, there is experimental, clinical, and molecular evidence suggesting keratoacanthoma is a distinct follicular neoplasm rather than a subtype of SCC.

4. Adenosquamous carcinoma should not be confused with cutaneous mucoepidermoid carcinoma or acantholytic SCC, both of which are less aggressive than adenosquamous carcinoma. Cutaneous mucoepidermoid carcinomas form goblet and intermediate cells without true glands. Acantholytic SCC is mucicarmine negative and forms pseudo-glands in nests of acantholytic tumor cells.

5. Bowen disease usually involves adnexal epithelium and may show extensive downward growth along adnexa, producing a thick neoplasm that extends deeply into the dermis. Bona fide invasive Bowen disease is very rare and requires unequivocal dermal invasion by tumor nests, not simply florid adnexal involvement.

14.4 Melanocytic Nevus

Melanocytic nevi are common benign cutaneous neoplasms comprised of melanocytes. They can be grouped into acquired, predominantly epidermal proliferations likely derived from epidermal melanocytic stem cells and congenital, predominantly dermal proliferations derived from dermal melanocytic stem cells [10]. Clark and coworkers described a subtype of melanocytic nevus, the dysplastic nevus, which they regarded as a precursor to melanoma [11]. The dysplastic nevus remains highly controversial. It is no longer considered a direct precursor to melanoma, though patients with a large number of dysplastic nevi are at higher risk for melanoma. Grading of atypia in dysplastic nevi is widespread, though it has been challenged on grounds of poor reproducibility, inconsistent criteria, and questionable significance [10, 11]. Proponents of grading atypia in dysplastic nevi cite studies demonstrating a higher incidence of a prior diagnosis of melanoma in patients with dysplastic nevi that sport high-grade atypia. Opponents of grading atypia note that many of the nuclear criteria used to denote high-grade atypia overlap with expected findings in Spitz, pleomorphic, and senescent nevi. Assessment of atypia in dysplastic nevi is a personal choice, though for those that opt to do so, a two-tiered system is probably more meaningful and reproducible than a three-tiered grading system. High-grade atypia should not be used as a crutch for cases in which the pathologist is unsure whether a melanocytic neoplasm is benign or malignant. In such cases, an expert opinion may be required, particularly if the lesion is >1 mm thick or forms dermal mitoses or expansile dermal nests.

- *Dysplastic nevus with low-grade atypia.* This melanocytic nevus (also known as Clark nevus) is comprised of melanocytes (Fig. 14.10). Some of these melanocytes have nuclei larger than those of nearby keratinocytes. They exhibit

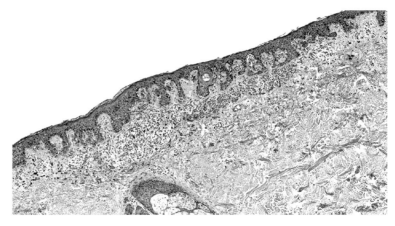

Fig. 14.10 Dysplastic/Clark nevus is a superficial proliferation of melanocytes with broad intraepidermal "shoulders" of melanocytes that often extend beyond a minor central dermal component, elongated rete ridges that may be fused, and periretal fibrosis, inflammation, and telangiectasias

a mostly intraepidermal growth pattern with peripheral extension of the epidermal melanocytes three or more rete ridges beyond a central dermal complement of melanocytes ("shoulders"). There are elongated and interconnected rete ridges, usually with a preponderance of singly dispersed melanocytes which are aligned along the tips and edges of the rete ridges. There is relative sparing of the suprapapillary epidermal arcs, mild fibro-inflammatory expansion of the papillary dermis, and few dermal melanophages.

- *Dysplastic nevus with high-grade atypia.* This diagnosis is used for melanocytic nevi with the above features and three or more of the following nuclear abnormalities: threefold variation in size (anisokaryosis), prominent nucleoli, hyperchromatism, and/or irregular membranes.

14.4.1 Comments

1. A grading system for atypical Spitz tumors in children and adolescents has been proposed [12, 13]. Spitz tumors can be divided into low-, intermediate-, and high-risk groups by a point system based on age at diagnosis greater than 10 years, tumor surface diameter greater than 10 mm, ulceration, involvement of the subcutaneous panniculus, and ≥ 6 mitoses/mm^2. Increasing risk is correlated with likelihood of lymph node involvement. However, the great majority of children with atypical Spitz tumors and nodal metastases do not exhibit progressive disease or fatal outcomes, and the significance of a positive lymph node in these patients is controversial.

14.5 Melanoma

Melanoma is a malignant neoplasm of melanocytes. It is estimated that approximately 70,000 individuals in the United States will be diagnosed with invasive melanoma in 2012 and that approximately 8,800 individuals will die of melanoma in 2012. Most melanomas can be subclassified as lentigo maligna melanoma, superficial spreading

melanoma, acral lentiginous melanoma, and nodular melanoma [14–18]. Melanoma subtypes do not have independent prognostic significance and are generally not utilized in therapeutic decision-making. However, some investigators have found differences in growth rates, and melanoma subtype may be a surrogate for tumor grade.

14.5.1 Subtypes of Melanoma

- *Lentigo maligna melanoma (extremely low grade).* Including in situ forms of melanoma, lentigo maligna melanoma comprises approximately 55 % of all melanomas. The median age of onset is in the eighth decade and there is a predilection for chronically sun-exposed sites such as the face. It is defined histopathologically by a preponderance of small, singly dispersed hyperchromic melanocytes with a propensity for growth along adnexa, effacement of the rete ridge pattern, and signs of sun damage such as solar elastosis and epidermal atrophy (Fig. 14.11).
- *Acral lentiginous melanoma (low grade).* It comprises 3 % of melanomas. Approximately 10–20 % of these tumors are associated with *c-KIT* gene mutations. They are located on acral skin and represent the most common form of melanoma in patients with skin of color. They are characterized by a proliferation of small melanocytes with angulated hyperchromic nuclei along the dermoepidermal junction (Fig. 14.12). The proliferation is often associated with an obscuring lymphocytic infiltrate, acanthosis, and extension of malignant cells along sweat ducts.
- *Superficial spreading melanoma (intermediate grade).* These tumors account for approximately 30 % of all skin melanomas and they often have *BRAF* gene mutations. Median age of onset is in the fifth decade and there is a predilection for intermittently sun-exposed sites such as the trunk and extremities. Histopathologically they are defined by scattering of enlarged melanocytes in the spinous layer of the epidermis and an intraepithelial complement of malignant melanocytes that extends at least 3 rete ridges beyond any dermal complement of malignant melanocytes (Fig. 14.13).

Fig. 14.11 Lentigo maligna melanoma is a relatively indolent form of melanoma that usually remains confined to the epidermis and is comprised of mostly singly dispersed small hyperchromic melanocytes in sun-damaged skin

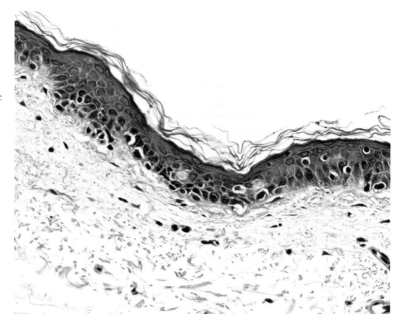

Fig. 14.12 Acral lentiginous melanoma is also comprised of singly dispersed hyperchromic melanocytes, but unlike lentigo maligna melanoma, the epidermis is thickened, sun damage is absent, and they are limited to acral skin

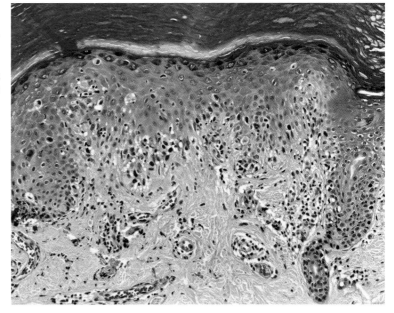

- *Nodular melanoma (high grade).* These tumors account for 4 % of all skin melanomas. Their median age of onset is in the seventh decade. Their distribution is random and not correlated with sun exposure. Malignant melanocytes typically form a dermal nodule (Fig. 14.14). Malignant melanocytes do not extend laterally beyond three rete ridges to either side of the nodule. Malignant epidermal melanocytes may be absent in so-called primary dermal melanomas.

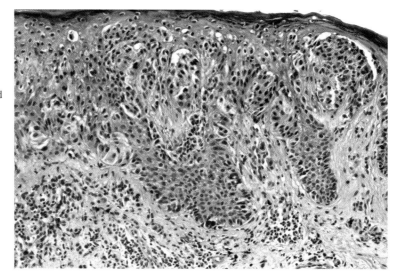

Fig. 14.13 Superficial spreading melanoma is comprised of epithelioid melanocytes, often with abundant melanin pigment. Malignant melanocytes are arranged in nests and scattered in the spinous layer of the epidermis

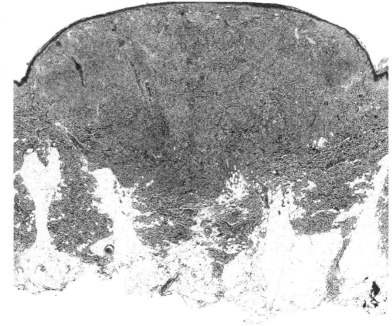

Fig. 14.14 Nodular melanoma forms a symmetric nodule centered in the dermis and involving the epidermis secondarily. Epidermal melanoma cells do not extend more than three rete ridges to either side of the dermal melanoma cells

14.5.2 Comments

1. Though prognosis is largely based on tumor thickness, dermal mitoses, and ulceration, subtype of melanoma is a required element in tumor checklists sponsored by the College of American Pathologists.

2. Rare melanoma subtypes include desmoplastic, nevoid, Spitzoid, mucosa, and childhood melanoma and melanoma arising in a blue or congenital nevus.

3. The desmoplastic subtype has bearing on prognosis and treatment. Pure desmoplastic melanomas behave more like sarcomas and

tend to metastasize hematogenously rather than via the lymphatic system. Hence, sentinel lymph node biopsy is not usually offered for pure desmoplastic melanoma, but postoperative radiotherapy may be beneficial.

Books and Monographs

LeBoit PE, Burg G, Weedon D, Sarasin A (eds) (2006) World Health Organization classification of tumors: pathology and genetics- skin tumors. IARC Press, Lyon

Weedon D (2010) Skin pathology, 3rd edn. Elsevier, China

Articles

1. Kaur P, Mulvaney M, Carlson JA (2006) Basal cell carcinoma progression correlates with host immune response and stromal alterations: a histologic analysis. Am J Dermatopathol 28:293–307
2. Cassarino DS, DeRienzo DP, Barr RJ (2006) Cutaneous squamous cell carcinoma: a comprehensive classification (part 1). J Cutan Pathol 33:191–206
3. Cassarino DS, DeRienzo DP, Barr RJ (2006) Cutaneous squamous cell carcinoma: a comprehensive classification (part 2). J Cutan Pathol 33:261–279
4. Kane CL, Keehn CA, Smithberger E, Glass LF (2004) Histopathology of cutaneous squamous cell carcinoma and its variants. Semin Cutan Med Surg 23:54–61
5. Khanna M, Fortier-Riberdy G, Smoller B, Dinehart S (2002) Reporting tumor thickness for cutaneous squamous cell carcinoma. J Cutan Pathol 29:321–323
6. Petter G, Haustein UF (2000) Histologic subtyping and malignancy assessment of cutaneous squamous cell carcinoma. Dermatol Surg 26:521–530
7. Sulica VI, Kao G (1988) Squamous-cell carcinoma of the scalp arising in lesions of discoid lupus erythematosus. Am J Dermatopathol 10:137–141
8. Breuninger H, Schaumburg-Lever G, Holzschuh J, Horny HP (1997) Desmoplastic squamous cell carcinoma of the skin and vermilion surface: a highly malignant subtype of skin cancer. Cancer 79:915–919
9. Jo VY, Fletcher CD (2011) p63 immunohistochemical staining is limited in soft tissue tumors. Am J Clin Pathol 136:762–766
10. Pozo L, Naase M, Cerio R et al (2001) Critical analysis of histologic criteria for grading atypical (dysplastic) nevi. Am J Clin Pathol 115:194–204
11. Clark WH Jr, Reimer RR, Greene M et al (1978) Origin of familial malignant melanomas from heritable melanocytic lesions. "The B-K mole syndrome". Arch Dermatol 114:732–738
12. Spatz A, Calonje E, Handfield-Jones S, Barnhill RL (1999) Spitz tumors in children: a grading system for risk stratification. Arch Dermatol 135:282–285
13. Ludgate MW, Fullen DR, Lee J et al (2009) The atypical Spitz tumor of uncertain biologic potential: a series of 67 patients from a single institution. Cancer 115:631–641
14. Forman SB, Ferringer TC, Peckham SJ et al (2008) Is superficial spreading melanoma still the most common form of malignant melanoma? J Am Acad Dermatol 58:1013–1020
15. Scolyer RA, Long GV, Thompson JF (2011) Evolving concepts in melanoma classification and their relevance to multidisciplinary melanoma patient care. Mol Oncol 5:124–136
16. Liu W, Dowling JP, Murray WK et al (2006) Rate of growth in melanomas: characteristics and associations of rapidly growing melanomas. Arch Dermatol 142:15551–15558
17. Lipsker D (2006) Growth rate, early detection, and prevention of melanoma: melanoma epidemiology revisited and future challenges. Arch Dermatol 142:1638–1640
18. Zalaudek I, Marghoob AA, Scope A et al (2008) Three roots of melanoma. Arch Dermatol 144:1375–1379

Tumors of the Central Nervous System

15

Muchou Joe Ma

15.1 Introduction

The first significant histologic classification of tumors of the central nervous system (CNS) was proposed by Bailey and Cushing in 1926. Thereafter, several major revisions were introduced, and numerous consensus conferences were held. The grading of CNS tumors is an integral part of these revisions and is routinely applied to primary intracranial and spinal tumors. The most widely accepted grading system is the World Health Organization (WHO) classification of tumors, last updated in 2007. Recently the prognostic values of several genetic markers have been validated in several CNS tumors, and the importance of testing them in paraffin-embedded tissue is growing [1]. Rare tumors, lymphomas, paraganglioma, and pituitary adenomas will not be discussed in this concise chapter.

15.2 Astrocytoma

Diffusely infiltrating or fibrillary astrocytomas constitute the majority of those encountered in the human central nervous system. The WHO classification determines the grade, on a scale of I–IV, of a diffusely infiltrating astrocytoma according to several microscopic features: cellularity, nuclear atypia, mitotic activity, vascular proliferation, and tumor necrosis. However, grading based on these criteria has been reported to show poor interobserver agreement, especially in stereotactic biopsies [2]. In 1988, Daumas-Duport and colleagues proposed a more reproducible grading system of adult diffusely infiltrating astrocytomas [3], generally known as the St. Anne/Mayo grading system. Assigning equal importance to each of four specific pathologic features – nuclear atypia, mitosis, vascular proliferation, and necrosis – the St. Anne/Mayo grade of a diffusely infiltrating astrocytoma on a scale of 1–4 is determined by the number of feature(s) present plus 1. This system is similar, but not identical to, the WHO classification. For instance, finding one mitotic figure in an otherwise well-differentiated, diffusely infiltrating astrocytoma qualifies it as grade 3 in the St. Anne/Mayo system, but it may still be considered a WHO grade II lesion. On the other hand, a small biopsy showing predominantly necrosis rimmed by a few viable atypical astrocytes without mitosis is diagnosed as glioblastoma (grade IV) by the WHO criteria but remains a St. Anne/Mayo grade 3 lesion. Since both systems are defined by positive features, grading fibrillary astrocytomas based on small biopsies is subject to errors of "undergrading."

The WHO classification of astrocytic tumors includes the following:

- Grade I, fibrillary astrocytoma. This tumor is exceedingly rare. It shows a mild increase of cellularity and minimal cytologic atypia

M.J. Ma, M.D., Ph.D.
Department of Pathology (Center for Diagnostic Pathology), Florida Hospital Orlando, 2855 North Orange Avenue, 32804 Orlando, FL, USA
e-mail: joe.ma.md@flhosp.org

I. Damjanov, F. Fan (eds.), *Cancer Grading Manual*,
DOI 10.1007/978-3-642-34516-6_15, © Springer-Verlag Berlin Heidelberg 2013

Fig. 15.1 Astrocytoma. This WHO grade II diffusely infiltrating fibrillary astrocytoma shows mild hypercellularity and mild nuclear atypia

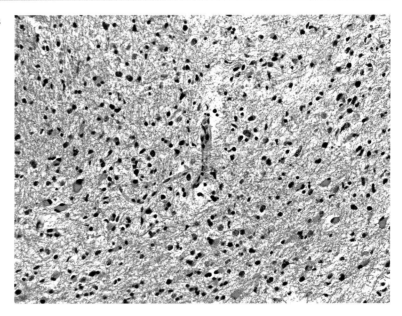

Fig. 15.2 Gemistocytic astrocytoma. This WHO grade II tumor has moderate atypia with a deceiving lack of detectable mitotic activity (luxol fast blue/HE stain)

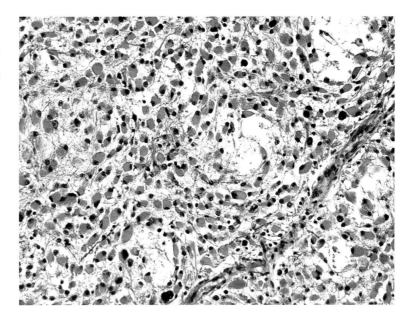

without other pathologic features. This grade also includes variants of astrocytoma with specific pathology, radiology, and indolent clinical behavior, i.e., pilocytic astrocytoma and subependymal giant cell astrocytoma.

• Grade II, well-differentiated or diffuse astrocytoma. This tumor shows a mild to moderate increase of cellularity and nuclear atypia (Fig. 15.1), minimal mitotic activity (usually <2 mitoses per tumor), and no vascular prolif-

eration or tumor necrosis. One variant of WHO grade II diffuse astrocytomas is gemistocytic astrocytoma that has been reported to portend a more aggressive behavior than its lack of mitotic activity suggests. It is composed of neoplastic astrocytes with eccentric nuclei, small nucleoli, and plump, eosinophilic, glassy, and fibrillary cytoplasm with frequent perivascular inflammation and no mitotic figures (Fig. 15.2).

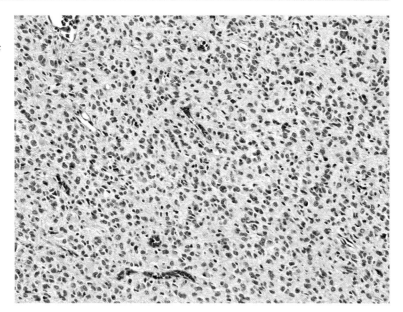

Fig. 15.3 Anaplastic astrocytoma. Moderate hypercellularity and cytologic atypia are seen in this WHO grade III tumor

- Grade III, anaplastic or malignant astrocytoma. This tumor has moderate to high cellularity (Fig. 15.3), prominent nuclear atypia, and readily identified mitotic figures. When neither tumor necrosis nor vascular proliferation is recognized, the distinction between grade II and grade III astrocytoma may be subjective. Mitotic count has been the most reliable criterion, with two or more mitoses found per microscopic section in grade III astrocytoma. The use of the MIB-1 labeling index to differentiate more aggressive astrocytomas from less aggressive ones has been suggested [4]; however, result of a recent study [5], significant overlap, and topographic variation of staining limit its practical use, especially in small specimens.
- Grade IV, glioblastoma. This group of tumors includes astrocytomas that not only show nuclear atypia but also exhibit either necrosis (pseudopalisaded or not) (Fig. 15.4) or vascular proliferation (Fig. 15.5) or both. As the old term glioblastoma multiforme implies, the architectural pattern and cytologic details of neoplastic cells are variable. Small cells, clear cells, giant cells with bizarre hyperchromatic nuclei, cells with eosinophilic granular cytoplasm, and spindled cells in fascicles can be seen in various combinations or, less often, in

pure forms. Aberrant epithelial (squamous and/or glandular) differentiation is rarely seen in glioblastomas and should not to be mistaken as collision cancer (carcinoma metastatic to glioblastoma), which occurs very rarely. Gliosarcoma is WHO grade IV tumor containing a glioblastoma component and a malignant mesenchymal component derived from vessel walls or associated meninges (Fig. 15.6).

15.2.1 Special Variants of Astrocytoma

In addition to the common variety of infiltrating astrocytomas, several other forms are recognized, including:
- Pilocytic astrocytoma (PA). The WHO grade I pilocytic astrocytoma is often cystic with an enhanced mural nodule. It is usually well circumscribed but may show microscopic infiltration in the surrounding parenchyma. It often occurs in or near the midline of neuraxis (e.g., cerebellum, hypothalamus, optic nerve) in children and young adults, but cases have been observed in all age groups and at all anatomic locations. The microscopic appearance of PA varies tremendously. Classic features include a biphasic growth pattern (fibrillary compact areas containing piloid cells and

Fig. 15.4 Glioblastoma. This WHO grade IV tumor shows characteristic pseudopalisaded necrosis

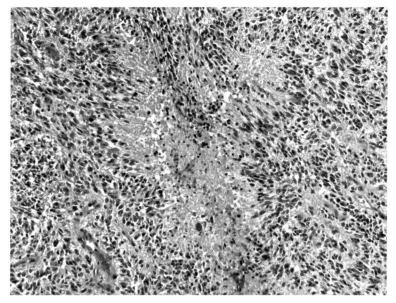

Fig. 15.5 Glioblastoma. Characteristic vascular proliferation is evident in this WHO grade IV tumor

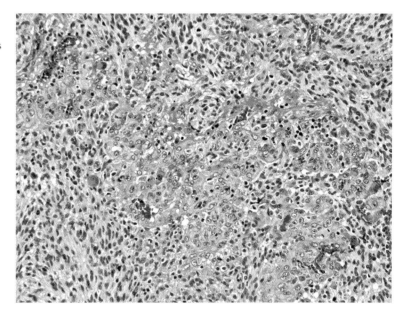

fibrillary processes with or without Rosenthal fibers, alternating with loose microcystic areas containing protoplasmic astrocytes in loose mucin [Fig. 15.7]), uniform cells, bland nuclei, eosinophilic granular bodies (Fig. 15.8), bipolar slender fibrillary cytoplasmic processes, and calcospherites. Other characteristics include a mild degree of cellular pleomorphism, nuclear atypia, giant cells with floret-like nuclei, hyalinized blood vessels, perinuclear halos, leptomeningeal infiltration, central infarctive necrosis, vascular proliferation, and palisaded spongioblastoma-like growth pattern. By themselves, necrosis and vascular proliferation are of no prognostic significance. In general, mitotic figures are rare and the MIB-1 labeling index is low (<4 %). Very rare cases of cerebellar PA with malignant features have been reported (WHO grade III) with hypercellularity, high mitotic

Fig. 15.6 Gliosarcoma. This WHO grade IV tumor contains GFAP-negative, atypical mesenchymal cells embedded in massive hyalinized stroma

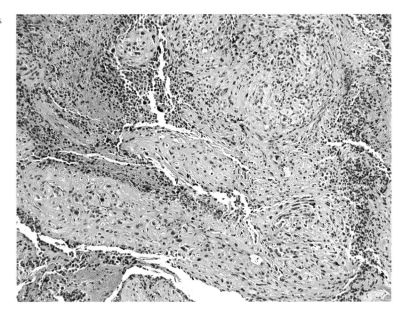

Fig. 15.7 Pilocytic astrocytoma. This WHO grade I tumor shows a fibrillary and loose microcystic biphasic growth pattern

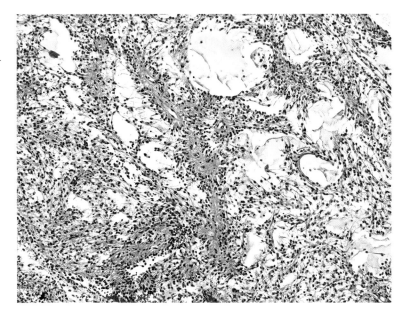

activity, and pseudopalisaded tumor necrosis [6]. Rarely, a PA may undergo malignant transformation after irradiation, with characteristics of WHO grade III–IV anaplastic astrocytoma or glioblastoma.

• Subependymal giant cell astrocytoma (SEGA). This WHO grade I circumscribed ventricular wall tumor is found either incidentally or after presentation with obstructive hydrocephalus. The majority of patients with this tumor have

tuberous sclerosis; 6–16 % of patients with this disease develop SEGA. Classic features include a loose or packed collection of large polygonal or elongated cells, with plump or fibrillary eosinophilic cytoplasm in between hyalinized blood vessels (with or without perivascular pseudopalisading) and calcospherites. Some polygonal cells may contain large, round to oval, and ganglionic (neuronal) nuclei with a single, central prominent nucleoli

Fig. 15.8 Pilocytic astrocytoma. Numerous eosinophilic granular bodies can be observed in this WHO grade I tumor

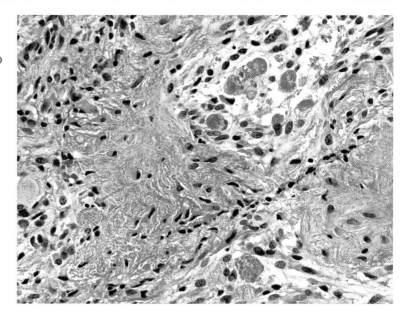

Fig. 15.9 Subependymal giant cell astrocytoma. In this WHO grade I tumor, large neoplastic cells are seen, with round nuclei, central prominent nucleoli, plump eosinophilic cytoplasm, and occasional multinucleation

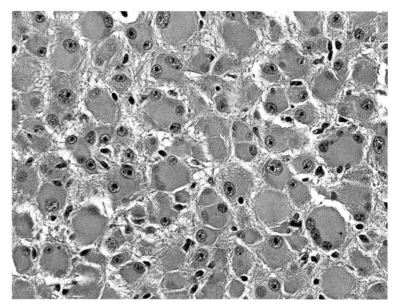

(Fig. 15.9). Mild cellular pleomorphism, binucleation, and occasional mitoses may be seen, but tumor necrosis and vascular proliferation are rare and do not portend malignancy.

- Pleomorphic xanthoastrocytoma (PXA). This WHO grade II tumor usually presents as a circumscribed, often partially cystic, superficial cerebral tumor in children and young adults. Characteristic features include elongated astrocytes, scattered giant cells with large

hyperchromatic nuclei, intranuclear pseudoinclusions, vacuolated (lipidized) cytoplasm (Fig. 15.10), scattered eosinophilic granular bodies, perivascular inflammation, and pericellular deposition of reticulin fibers. Most cases are controlled or cured by complete surgical resection. A minority (15–20 %) of PXA manifest tumor necrosis, vascular proliferation, and a higher mitotic activity (>5 mitoses per 10 hpf). These so-called PXA with

Fig. 15.10 Pleomorphic xanthoastrocytoma. Large cells with bizarre hyperchromatic nuclei, intranuclear pseudoinclusions, and vacuolated cytoplasm are hallmarks of this WHO grade II tumor

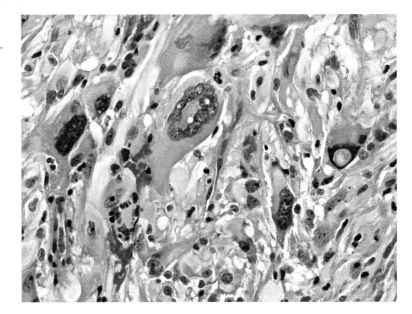

Fig. 15.11 Desmoplastic infantile ganglioglioma. This WHO grade I tumor consists of neoplastic astrocytes with plump fibrillary cytoplasm embedded in sclerotic stroma

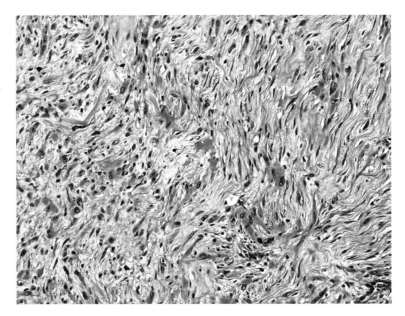

anaplastic features may have a less favorable prognosis [7]; however, they should not be confused with giant cell glioblastoma.

- Desmoplastic cerebral astrocytoma of infancy (DCAI) and desmoplastic infantile ganglioglioma (DIGG). These rare WHO grade I massive neoplasms of young children present as large, solid, and cystic cerebral tumors often associated with the dura and leptomeninges. Microscopically, desmoplastic hypocellular zones containing plump fibrillary astrocytes (Fig. 15.11) transform to hypercellular zones of round or spindled cells with atypia and high nucleocytoplasmic ratios (Fig. 15.12). In spite of the readily found mitotic figures and their alarming size, these neoplasms have a good prognosis following resection. The histopathologies of both are similar, except for the presence of small or large cells with neuronal differentiation in DIGG.

Fig. 15.12 Desmoplastic infantile ganglioglioma. Some areas of this WHO grade I tumor are variably hypercellular and contain small cells with oval or elongated nuclei and scant cytoplasm

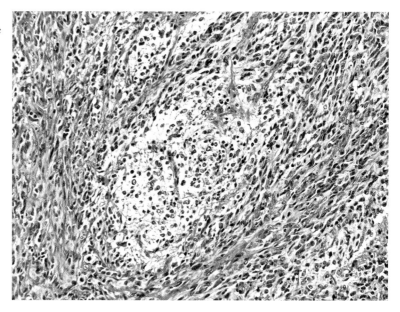

- Rare variants of astrocytoma. This heterogeneous group, not discussed here, includes several entities: protoplasmic astrocytoma, gliomatosis cerebri, chordoid glioma of the third ventricle, granular cell astrocytoma, astroblastoma, pilomyxoid astrocytoma of the suprasellar region in young children and infants, angiocentric glioma, gliofibroma, and sarcoglioma. For grading and characteristic features of these tumors, see specialized neuropathology textbooks and original articles.

15.3 Oligodendroglioma

The WHO classification recognizes two grades of oligodendroglioma: well-differentiated (WHO grade II) and anaplastic (malignant) (WHO grade III). It should be noted that clinical response of many oligodendrogliomas to certain chemotherapeutic agents – such as a PCV regimen (procarbazine, lomustine or CCNU, vincristine) and temozolomide – has been associated with codeletions of chromosomes 1p and 19q found in up to 80 % of grade II and up to two-thirds of grade III oligodendrogliomas.

- WHO grade II, well-differentiated oligodendroglioma. The classic features of well-

differentiated oligodendroglioma include superficial parenchymal (cortical) involvement, infiltrative borders, uniform cells with round nuclei and perinuclear halos (Fig. 15.13), scant cytoplasm without processes, or globular eccentric eosinophilic cytoplasm with fibrillary processes (mini- or microgemistocytes) (Fig. 15.14), a delicate capillary network, associated calcospherites, mucinous microcysts, and occasional hypercellular nodules. Marked nuclear atypia and occasional mitoses may be present. As in infiltrating astrocytomas, mitotic activity has been proposed as a major grading criterion with most grade II lesions showing less than 6 mitoses per 10 hpf [8] and MIB-1 labeling index of <5 %.

- WHO grade III, anaplastic or malignant oligodendroglioma. In addition to the features described above, this tumor shows diffuse hypercellularity, nuclear atypia, cellular pleomorphism, and brisk mitotic activity (Fig. 15.15). Vascular proliferation and tumor necrosis (with or without pseudopalisading) may be observed (Fig. 15.16), but neither feature is a necessary criterion. Some cases may display marked cellular pleomorphism and the formation of giant or elongated

Fig. 15.13 Oligodendroglioma. This WHO grade II tumor has uniform neoplastic cells with round nuclei and perinuclear halos between delicate capillaries

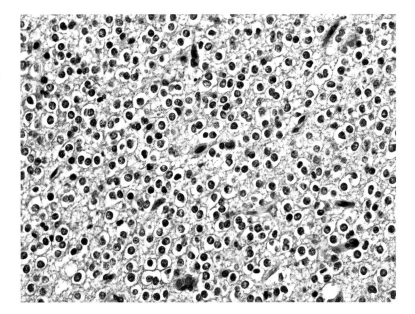

Fig. 15.14 Oligodendroglioma. This WHO grade II tumor contains areas of mini- or microgemistocytes

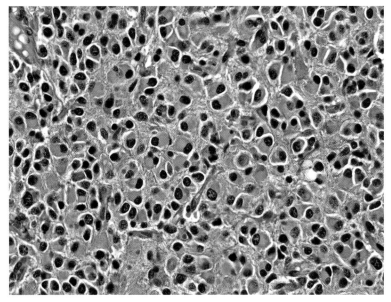

cells, making recognition of oligodendrocytic differentiation and distinction from astrocytomas difficult and subjective. Mixed oligoastrocytomas are diagnostic challenges in both classification and grading. A study has concluded that the identification of even a minor (100× microscopic field) component of oligodendroglioma imparts a better prognosis than a pure astrocytoma of the same grade [9]. Since there is no grade IV oligodendroglioma, distinction between anaplastic oligodendroglioma, anaplastic oligoastrocytoma, and glioblastoma can be arbitrary. An alternative is to classify it as WHO grade IV glioblastoma with an oligodendroglioma component, the prognosis of which appears better than that of conventional glioblastoma [10].

Fig. 15.15 Anaplastic oligodendroglioma. This WHO grade III tumor displays nuclear atypia and a brisk mitotic activity

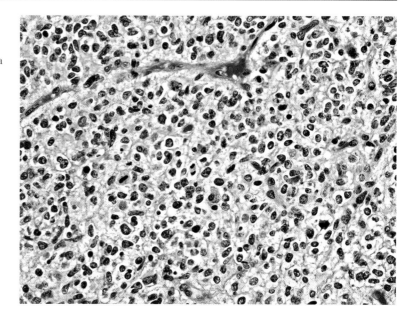

Fig. 15.16 Anaplastic oligodendroglioma. Vascular proliferation and necrosis are sufficient but not necessary features in this WHO grade III tumor

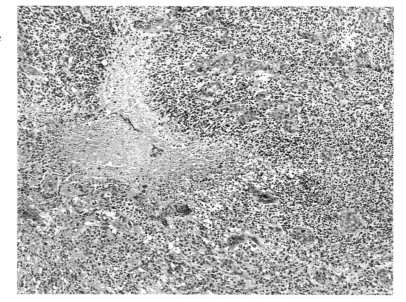

15.4   Ependymoma

Ependymoma arises from ependymal cells lining the cerebrospinal fluid pathways. This tumor occurs in any age group and is found often in the posterior fossa of children and young adults. The WHO classification recognizes several subtypes, graded on a scale from I to III, as follows:

• WHO grade I subependymoma. This group comprises nodular, well-demarcated, and fibrillary ependymal neoplasms on the walls of ventricles and the central canal (spinal cord). Microscopically, subependymomas are paucicellular and fibrillary, with the formation of microcysts and hyalinized vessels. Neoplastic cells are uniform in size and shape, with small round to oval nuclei, vacuolated or eosinophilic cytoplasm (Fig. 15.17) and tend to be clustered. Scattered cells with large pleomorphic nuclei of a degenerative nature and

Fig. 15.17 Subependymoma. In this WHO grade I tumor, cytologically bland cells and associated microcysts are observed in fibrillary matrix

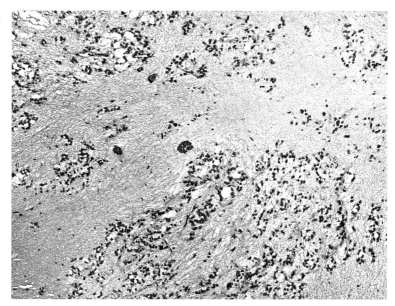

Fig. 15.18 Myxopapillary ependymoma. This WHO grade I tumor contains mucinous pools. The papillary growth pattern is a hallmark of this tumor

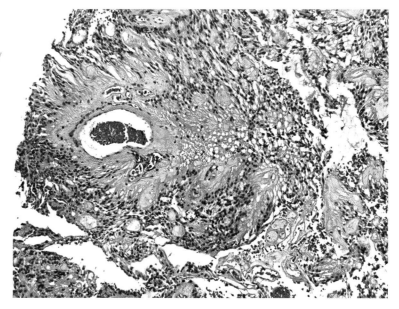

occasional mitoses may be seen, but necrosis and vascular proliferation is absent. Rare cases of WHO grade II mixed subependymoma and ependymoma containing features of both have been reported.

- WHO grade I myxopapillary ependymoma. This tumor is almost exclusively found in the conus medullaris/cauda equina region of young adults. Radially arranged, uniform, cuboidal, or elongated glial cells line the sur-

face of papillae with vascular, hyalinized, or myxoid cores (Fig. 15.18). Mucinous vacuoles or microcysts exist between cells. Mitotic activity is low. Local recurrence after resection is uncommon.

- WHO grade II ependymoma. This often demarcated glial neoplasm shows ependymal differentiation, evidenced by cellular uniformity, varying amounts of fibrillary cytoplasm, and the formation of perivascular

Fig. 15.19 Ependymoma.
Cells forming perivascular
pseudorosettes comprise this
WHO grade II tumor

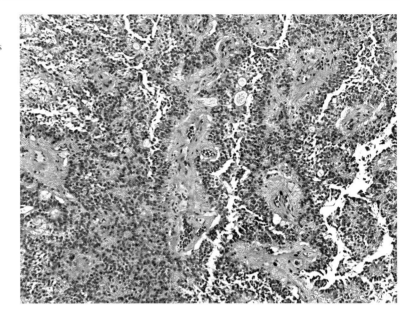

Fig. 15.20 Ependymoma.
This area of the WHO
grade II tumor contains an
ependymal canal

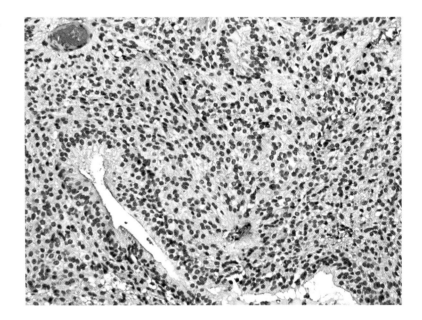

pseudorosettes (Fig. 15.19) and true ependymal rosettes (also known as ependymal
canals) (Fig. 15.20). The borders are pushing or, less commonly, infiltrative. In general
mitotic activity is low. Cystic change, stromal
hyalinization, and calcification may be present. Observed multiple patterns of growth
and cytology have given rise to four subtypes
recognized by WHO: cellular ependymoma,

clear cell ependymoma (Fig. 15.21), papillary
ependymoma, and tanycytic ependymoma.
Features of two or more of these subtypes may
be seen focally in a given case, so a subtype is
designated only when a pattern predominates
(>50 % of the areas examined).
• WHO grade III (anaplastic or malignant)
ependymoma. In addition to ependymal differentiation, this tumor shows anaplastic features

Fig. 15.21 Clear cell ependymoma. Some cells of this WHO grade II tumor have clear cytoplasm

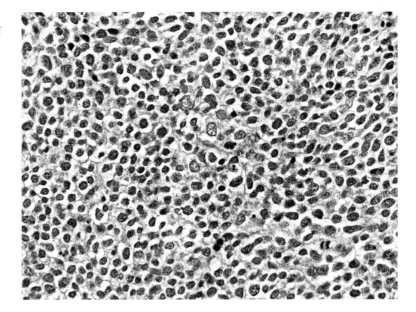

Fig. 15.22 Anaplastic ependymoma. Necrosis and vascular proliferation are evident in this tumor, as well as brisk mitotic activity and marked cytologic atypia

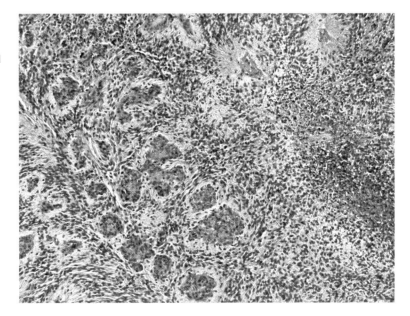

such as hypercellularity, cytologic anaplasia, brisk mitotic activity, pseudopalisaded necrosis, and vascular proliferation (Fig. 15.22). However, necrosis without palisading in a posterior fossa ependymoma is not diagnostic of anaplastic ependymoma. Pseudorosettes are inconspicuous, and true rosettes are hardly seen.

15.5   Embryonal Tumors, Neuronal Tumors, and Mixed Glioneuronal Tumors

When most constituents in a neuroepithelial neoplasm are poorly differentiated or undifferentiated, it is categorized as a WHO grade IV embryonal tumor or primitive neuroectodermal

Fig. 15.23 Medulloblastoma, classic type. The tumor cells form Homer-Wright (neuroblastic) rosettes

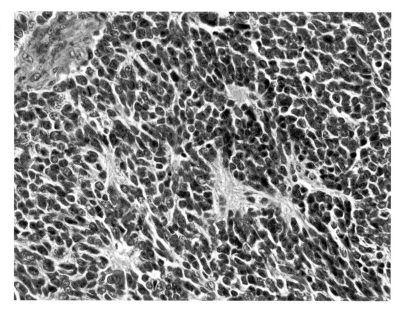

tumor (PNET). When found in the cerebellum, the pineal gland, and the posterior orbit, PNET is known as medulloblastoma, pineoblastoma, and retinoblastoma, respectively. A neuronal tumor consists of cells with neuronal (ganglionic or neurocytic) differentiation. They include WHO grade I neuronal hamartoma and gangliocytoma, and WHO grade II central (and extraventricular) neurocytoma. Neoplasms containing both mature neuronal and glial components are known as gangliogliomas or mixed glioneuronal tumors (e.g., papillary and rosette-forming variants, not discussed). Less frequently, a neuroepithelial neoplasm consists of a glial component – usually a diffusely infiltrating astrocytoma – and an embryonal component, without the formation of neurons or neurocytes. These are high-grade malignancies of WHO grade III to IV.

15.5.1 Medulloblastoma

These WHO grade IV embryonal neoplasms typically occur in the cerebellum (especially the vermis) of children and young adults. Like other PNET, medulloblastoma tends to spread through cerebrospinal fluid circulation and may metastasize to extraneural sites. Generally regarded as malignant, medulloblastomas show varying degrees of neuronal and glial differentiation in histopathology and immunohistochemistry. Four histologic subtypes are recognized (see below) with apparently different prognosis – patients with desmoplastic medulloblastomas and cerebellar neuroblastomas have a better prognosis than those with classic medulloblastomas, while those with large cell medulloblastomas have a worse prognosis.

- Classic medulloblastoma. This is the most common form. It consists of diffuse sheets of embryonic cells with round-, oval-, or carrot-shaped hyperchromatic nuclei and scant cytoplasm with possible formation of neuroblastic or Homer-Wright rosettes (Fig. 15.23) and astrocytic differentiation shown by glial fibrillary acidic protein (GFAP) expression. Pale areas of lower cellularity and containing cells with neuronal and astrocytic differentiation may be observed (Fig. 15.24). Neoplastic cells infiltrate the neural parenchyma at interface. Apoptotic bodies and mitotic figures vary in density.
- Desmoplastic (nodular) medulloblastoma. This tumor tends to be located in the cerebellar hemisphere rather than the vermis. It displays biphasic histology and contains many hypocellular, sometimes confluent nodules between reticulin-rich and hypercellular areas

Fig. 15.24 Medulloblastoma, classic type. In addition to undifferentiated cells, the tumor displays focal neuronal differentiation

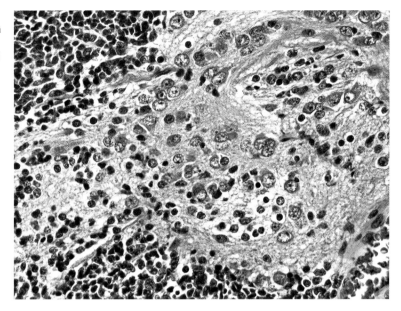

Fig. 15.25 Medulloblastoma, desmoplastic type. The tumor shows obvious nodularity

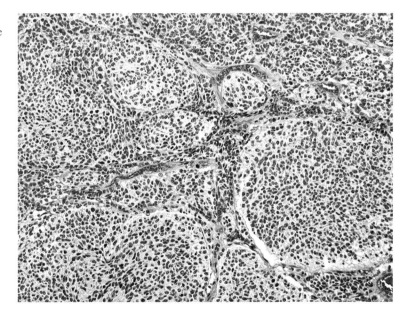

(Fig. 15.25). Cells in nodules are more differentiated (neuronal, neurocytic, and astrocytic), with uniform, round to oval nuclei of varying sizes embedded in a fibrillary, neuropil-like matrix.

• Medulloblastoma with extensive nodularity and advanced neuronal differentiation (cerebellar neuroblastoma). This rare tumor tends to occur in young children (usually <3 years of age). It

displays a strikingly lobular appearance on neuroimaging that corresponds to multiple large nodules on histology. Intranodular neoplastic cells have small, round nuclei and resemble those found in central neurocytomas, accompanied by occasional large neurons.

• Large cell (anaplastic) medulloblastoma. This tumor accounts for 5–25 % of all medulloblastomas. It consists of cells with large, round, or

Fig. 15.26 Medulloblastoma, large cell or anaplastic type. The tumor consists of cells with large, round, or pleomorphic vesicular nuclei showing molding or wrapping. The nucleoli are prominent and the cytoplasm more abundant than in classic medulloblastoma

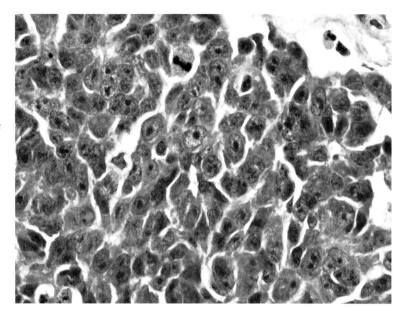

pleomorphic vesicular nuclei, prominent nucleoli, and abundant cytoplasm (Fig. 15.26). Frequently, there is nuclear molding, cell wrapping, necrosis, and high apoptotic and mitotic activities. Distinction from the highly malignant atypical teratoid/rhabdoid tumor (AT/RT, not discussed) in infants and young children may require the aid of immunohistochemistry.

15.5.2 Supratentorial Primitive Neuroepithelial Tumor

This WHO grade IV neoplasm also occurs in children and young adults with a histology (Fig. 15.27) similar to classic medulloblastoma. In general, their cells are poorly differentiated, but some may display divergent differentiation (e.g., neuroblastic, neuronal, astrocytic, ependymal, oligodendrocytic, muscular, and melanocytic). When both neuroblasts and differentiated neurons predominate, the terms cerebral neuroblastoma and ganglioneuroblastoma (Fig. 15.28) may be applied.

15.5.3 Pineal Parenchymal Tumor

The histopathologic hallmark of pineal parenchymal tumors is the pineocytomatous rosettes – small- to

medium-size, ill-defined zones of fibrillary processes rimmed by nuclei (Fig. 15.29). Pineocytomatous rosettes are larger and less regular in shape than Homer-Wright rosettes. These tumors include the following:

• Pineoblastoma. This WHO grade IV tumor is a poorly differentiated neoplasm in children showing high-grade features expected of PNET.
• Pineocytoma. This is a slow-growing WHO grade I tumor that affects young adults. It consists of sheets or lobules of small, uniform cells resembling normal pineocytes, arranged between small blood vessels (Fig. 15.30). Rarely, large- or medium-size ganglion cells and mitoses are found.
• Pineal parenchymal tumor of intermediate differentiation. This WHO grades II–III tumor shows signs of intermediate differentiation and has features that range between those of pineocytomas and pineoblastomas.

15.5.4 Gangliocytoma and Ganglioglioma

Gangliocytoma is a WHO grade I neoplasm of varying cellularity containing numerous differentiated ganglion cells (Fig. 15.31). Typically, this

Fig. 15.27 Supratentorial PNET. This WHO grade IV tumor shows histology identical to classic medulloblastoma

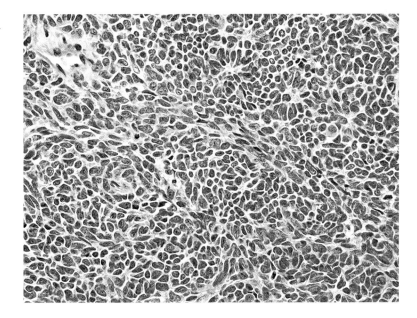

Fig. 15.28 Ganglioneuro-blastoma, WHO grade IV. The tumor is composed of well-differentiated (*right half*) and poorly differentiated (*left half*) areas

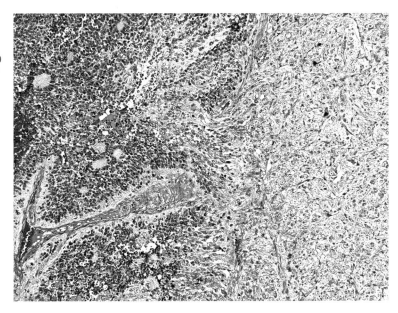

tumor contains hyalinized blood vessels with eosinophilic granular bodies, Rosenthal fibers, calcospherites, and perivascular inflammation. When both dysplastic neurons and neoplastic glia (usually astrocytes) are present, the neoplasm qualifies as a ganglioglioma. The glial component (astrocytic or oligodendrocytic) in a ganglioglioma determines its grade and behavior. It may be well differentiated similar to pilocytic astrocytoma (WHO grade I) (Fig. 15.32), anaplastic (WHO grade III), or, very rarely, indistinguishable from glioblastoma (WHO grade IV).

15.5.5 Central Neurocytoma

This sharply demarcated WHO grade II neoplasm is typically found in the lateral and third ventricles

Fig. 15.29 Pineocytoma. The tumor cells form pineocytomatous rosettes. These structures show vague circular, nuclear arrangements around fibrillary matrix and are larger than Homer-Wright rosettes

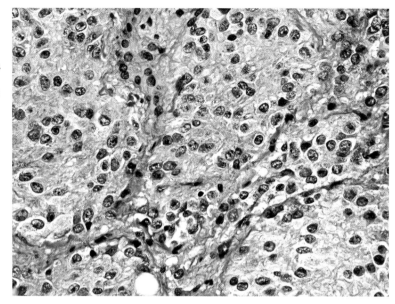

Fig. 15.30 Pineocytoma. The tumor has a lobular structure, and it is difficult at times to distinguish pineocytoma from the normal pineal gland

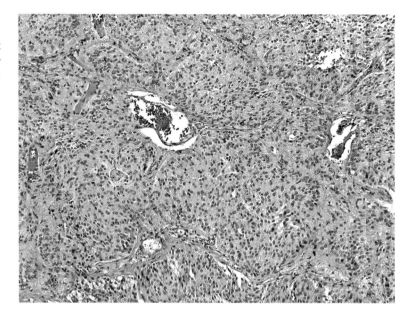

(near the foramen of Monro) of young adults. It consists of uniform round neoplastic neurocytes with small, round to oval nuclei and pale, granular, eosinophilic, or clear cytoplasm between delicate or hyalinized blood vessels and scattered calcospherites (Fig. 15.33). Isolated or small clusters of larger ganglionic cells and small, ill-defined, and neuropil-like fibrillary zones may be present. Strong synaptophysin and NeuN immunoreactivity is typical and helps its differentiation from oligodendroglioma. There are no histological prognosticators, except that a MIB-1 labeling index of >2–3 % has been associated with a shorter recurrence-free interval. Extraventricular locations and cases with anaplastic features (WHO grade III) have been reported [11].

Fig. 15.31 Gangliocytoma. Large dysplastic ganglion cells admixed with infiltrating lymphocytes and plasma cells are typical of these WHO grade I tumors

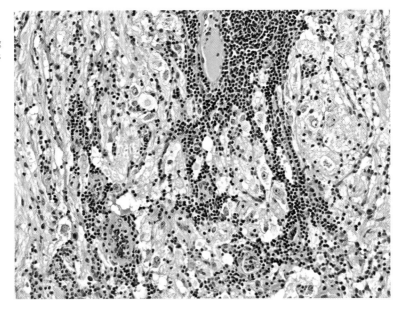

Fig. 15.32 Ganglioglioma. This WHO grade I tumor contains dysplastic neurons and atypical astrocytes

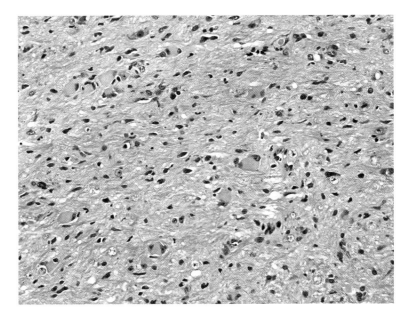

15.5.6 Dysembryoplastic Neuroepithelial Tumor (DNET)

This WHO grade I glioneuronal neoplasm occurs in children and young adults. It has a supratentorial cortical (especially the temporal lobe) location and is multinodular on neuroimaging and gross examination. Characteristic histology includes prominent nodular growth, a specific glioneuronal element (small oligodendrocyte-like cells decorating delicate columns of axons arranged perpendicular to the cortical surface), small mucinous cysts containing floating neurons, scattered stellate astrocytes with or without brown granular cytoplasmic pigment, and adjacent cortical dysplasia (Fig. 15.34). Rare tumors with identical histology have also been reported in the septum pellucidum and corpus callosum.

Fig. 15.33 Central neurocytoma. This WHO grade II neoplasm bears striking resemblance to oligodendroglioma

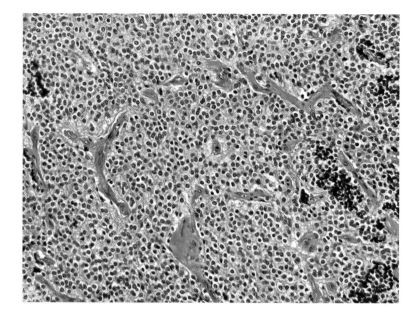

Fig. 15.34 Dysembryoplastic neuroepithelial tumor. This WHO grade I neoplasm contains uniform, bland, and oligodendrocyte-like cells between small mucinous cysts containing floating neurons

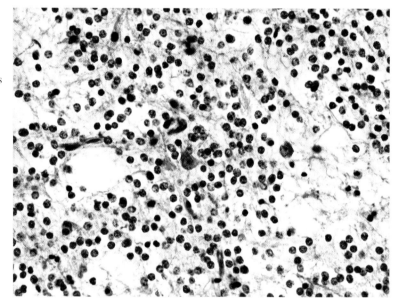

15.6   Meningioma

Meningioma is a neoplasm of meningothelial or arachnoid cap cells found in the leptomeninges. It is assigned WHO grades of I to III and is known to display widely variable histopathology. The list of recognized variants of meningiomas continues to change, and at least 13 were described in the 2007 WHO classification. Some variants occur in pure forms (e.g., secretory and clear cell meningiomas), while diagnostic features of others (e.g., chordoid, rhabdoid, and papillary meningiomas) are found only focally. It has been proposed that variant-specific features be observed in >50 % of tumor in order for its designation although this has yet to be accepted universally. WHO grade II atypical meningiomas have a higher risk for local recurrence and

Fig. 15.35 Brain-invasive meningioma. Fingerlike projections of neoplastic meningothelial cells into brain parenchyma without intervening leptomeninges are typical of this WHO grade II tumor

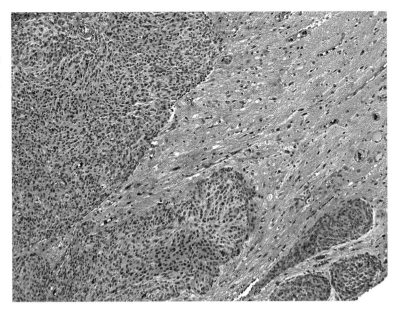

malignant transformation after resection/treatment, and WHO grade III malignant (anaplastic) meningiomas have the additional potential of cerebrospinal fluid seeding and distant metastasis. Invasion into the adjacent brain parenchyma may be observed in meningiomas of all grades and is an independent risk factor for local recurrence (hence, the assignment of brain-invasive meningiomas as WHO grade II). Brain invasion is evidenced by an irregular rather than smooth pushing border at the interface (without intervening leptomeninges), with small irregular nests or burrowing tongues of neoplastic meningothelial cells displaced in the parenchyma (Fig. 15.35).

15.6.1 WHO Grade I Benign Meningioma

This group of tumors includes several variants:
- Meningothelial or syncytial meningioma. Tumors of this group consist of neoplastic meningothelial cells with round, oval, or elongated nuclei, smooth nuclear profiles, dispersed chromatin, indistinct small nucleoli, and occasional intranuclear pseudoinclusions. Various architectural patterns and structures may be formed, most commonly whorls (Fig. 15.36) and syncytia (Fig. 15.37).
- Fibrous or fibroblastic meningioma. This tumor is composed of slender fibrocyte-like cells between collagen (Fig. 15.38).
- Psammomatous meningioma. Psammoma bodies are present in most meningiomas, but if they predominate over tumor cells in between, the tumor may be classified as a psammomatous meningioma.
- Secretory meningioma. This tumor has plump and epithelioid cells in sheets, forming scattered round vacuolar spaces that contain eosinophilic hyaline globules (pseudopsammoma bodies) (Fig. 15.39). Pericytic proliferation around blood vessels may be prominent. Surrounding brain parenchyma is often edematous.
- Angiomatous meningioma. Numerous, often hyalinized blood vessels between scarce neoplastic cells characterize this tumor (Fig. 15.40). It often coexists with microcystic change and may be associated with surrounding brain edema. It should not be confused with hemangioblastoma or meningeal hemangioma.
- Microcystic meningioma. This tumor consists of cells with thin elongated processes between clear or fluid-filled vacuoles and microcysts in a characteristic cobweb pattern (Fig. 15.41). Sometimes cells appear filled with small cytoplasmic vesicles that indent small or large

Fig. 15.36 Meningothelial meningioma. Tumor cells form whorls

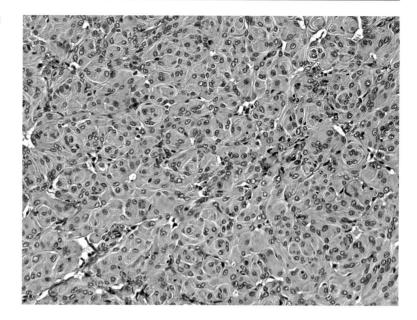

Fig. 15.37 Meningothelial meningioma. Streaming neoplastic meningothelial cells display oval nuclei and intranuclear pseudoinclusions in syncytia

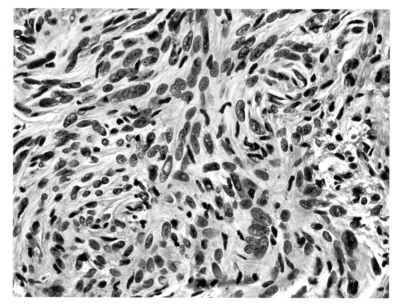

hyperchromatic nuclei. Abundant, often hyalinized, blood vessels are present. It should not be confused with clear cell meningioma.
- Lymphoplasmacyte-rich meningioma. In this rare variant, the tumor typically contains extensive infiltrates of chronic inflammatory cells.
- Metaplastic meningioma. This is a rare variant characterized by the formation of bone, cartilage, and/or apparent fat.

15.6.2 WHO Grade II Atypical Meningioma

According the WHO classification, a diagnosis of atypical meningioma should be made if the tumor has an average mitotic rate of ≥4 per 10 hpf or has three or more of the following five features: prominent nucleoli (Fig. 15.42); tumor necrosis; sheet-like, patternless growth; small cells with

Fig. 15.38 Fibrous meningioma. Elongated fibroblastic cells embedded in collagenous stroma comprise this tumor

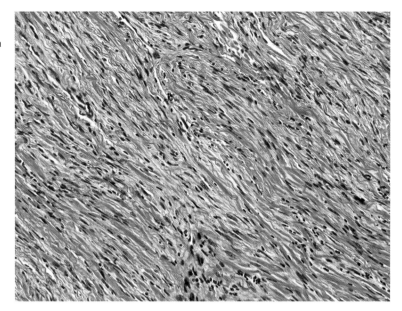

Fig. 15.39 Secretory meningioma. The tumor contains eosinophilic hyaline globules or "pseudopsammoma" bodies that are PAS positive and CEA immunoreactive

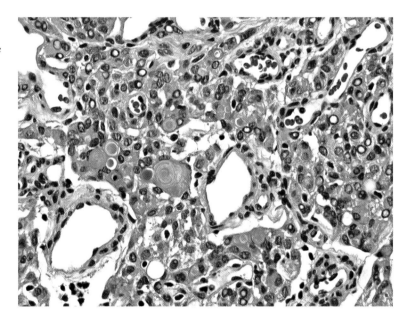

high nucleocytoplasmic ratios; and hypercellularity (Fig. 15.43). Of these features, only tumor necrosis is objective. Tumor necrosis in meningiomas appears as small or large areas of coagulative necrosis rimmed by a condensed band of cells. It should be distinguished from rare spontaneous central infarction and from infarctive necrosis resulting from presurgical embolization. Occasionally, neoplastic meningothelial cells have enlarged, hyperchromatic nuclei, but these changes are degenerative and are not indicative of true atypia. Two specific variants are designated WHO grade II, due to their atypical clinical behavior:

- Clear cell meningioma. This rare neoplasm is composed almost exclusively of clear cells with glycogen-rich cytoplasm and central small nuclei (Fig. 15.44). Numerous

Fig. 15.40 Angiomatous meningioma. The tumor is highly vascular and often contains cells with features of microcystic meningioma

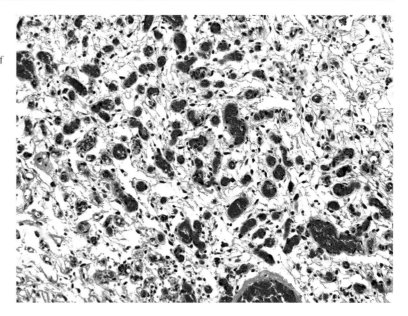

Fig. 15.41 Microcystic meningioma. Numerous small vacuoles and larger micro-cysts between cells typify this tumor – note the characteristic "cobweb" pattern of cytoplasmic processes and peripherally placed nuclei

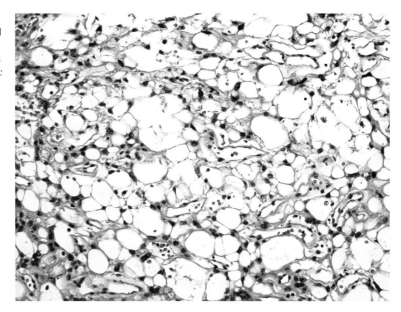

thick collagenous fibers and, sometimes, prominent hyalinization are found in the stroma. Whorls are not apparent, and psammoma bodies are rare. Many are found at the cerebellopontine angle or the cauda equina region in children and young adults. They have a high risk for cerebrospinal fluid seeding and local recurrence after initial treatment.

• Chordoid meningioma. This tumor is rarely found in a pure form. Typically, it is composed of anastomosing cords of epithelioid, sometimes vacuolated, neoplastic cells in a myxoid background (Fig. 15.45).

Fig. 15.42 Atypical meningioma. The WHO grade II tumor contains cells with prominent nucleoli

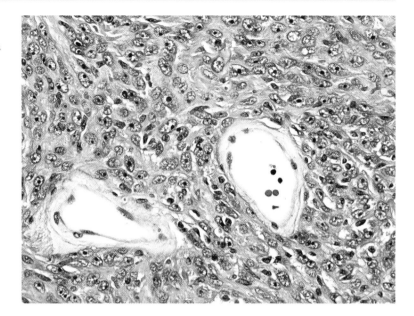

Fig. 15.43 Atypical meningioma. The tumor appears hypercellular because the small hyperchromatic cells have scant cytoplasm and are compacted into "patternless" sheets

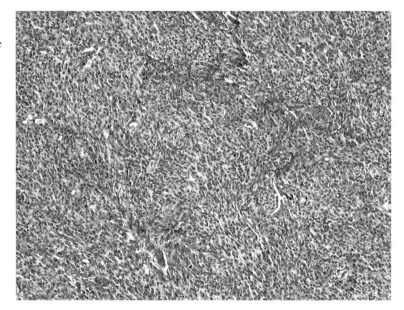

15.6.3 WHO Grade III, Malignant or Anaplastic Meningioma

This group includes meningothelial neoplasms with a very brisk mitotic rate (≥20 per 10 hpf) and other atypical features, or dura-based sarcoma without meningothelial or heterologous differentiation (meningeal sarcomas) (Fig. 15.46). The following two histological variants also are known to behave in a malignant fashion:

- Papillary meningioma. This tumor has a predilection for children and young adults. The hallmark of this neoplasm is the formation of perivascular pseudorosettes in discohesive

Fig. 15.44 Clear cell meningioma. This WHO grade II tumor is composed of bland cells with PAS-positive, diastase-sensitive clear cytoplasm and small, centrally located nuclei between "ropey" collagen

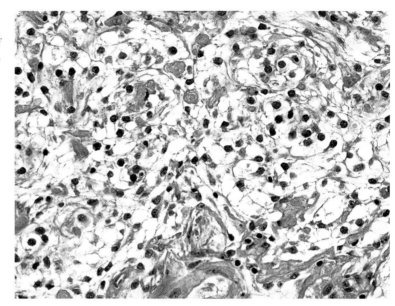

Fig. 15.45 Chordoid meningioma. The epithelioid tumor cells form inter-anastomosing cords in a myxoid background

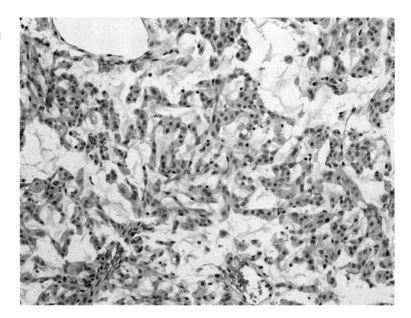

regions of the neoplasm (Fig. 15.47). Although neoplastic cells display bland cytology (Fig. 15.48), mitoses are readily found.

• Rhabdoid meningioma. This variant is rarely found in a pure form, and meningothelial whorls are seen focally. Rhabdoid cells have large vesicular and eccentric nuclei adjacent to globular cytoplasmic bodies composed of intermediate filaments (Fig. 15.49). They are either nested or found in massive sheets.

Fig. 15.46 Meningeal
sarcoma. Spindle-shaped
tumor cells show marked
atypia, a brisk mitotic activity,
and no meningothelial
differentiation

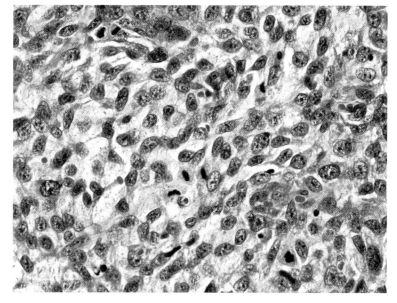

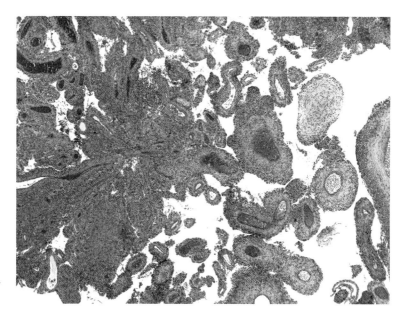

Fig. 15.47 Papillary
meningioma. The tumor cells
line the fibrovascular cores of
well-formed papillae

Fig. 15.48 Papillary meningioma. The papillae are lined by neoplastic cells that still have meningothelial features, such as intranuclear pseudoinclusions (*upper left*) and whorls (not shown)

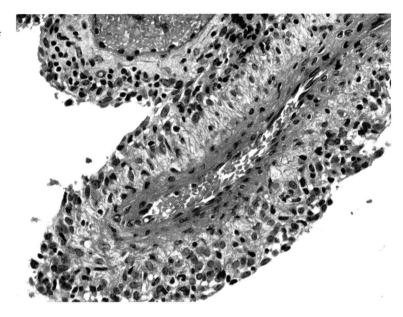

Fig. 15.49 Rhabdoid meningioma. The tumor cells have a well-developed cytoplasm that contains globular bodies and eccentric, frequently indented nuclei

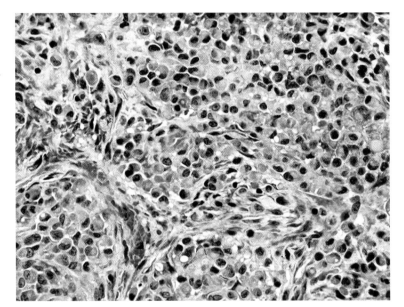

15.7 Choroid Plexus Neoplasm

Neoplasms of the choroid plexus epithelium are found in or adjacent to the ventricles, including the cerebellopontine angle. Calcification is common. They present a spectrum spanning from discrete and easily resected benign papillomas to infiltrative high-grade carcinomas with intermediate forms:

• Choroid plexus papilloma, WHO grade I. This benign neoplasm occurs in patients of all ages. Papillary fronds are lined by a single layer of cuboidal to columnar epithelia over fibrovascular cores. The nuclei of the epithelia are bland, and mitotic activity is low (Fig. 15.50). Focal cytoplasmic clearing may be present. Occasionally, small islands of glial tissue are incorporated in the papillary cores,

Fig. 15.50 Choroid plexus papilloma. This WHO grade I tumor is composed of cylindrical cells lining papillary structures

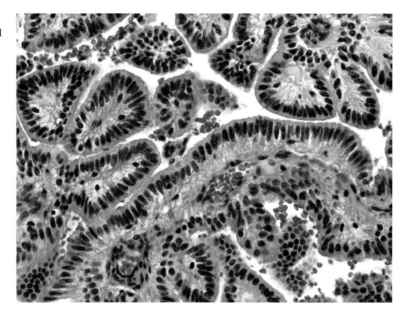

Fig. 15.51 Atypical choroid plexus papilloma. This WHO grade II papillary tumor shows hypercellularity and occasional mitotic figures (*right lower corner*)

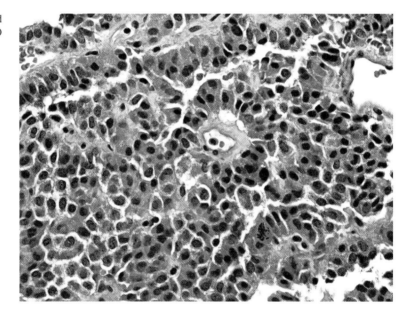

but brain invasion, cytologic anaplasia, and necrosis are not seen.

- Atypical choroid plexus papilloma, WHO grade II. This recently described [12] intermediate grade of choroid plexus neoplasms is defined by a mitotic count of ≥2 mitoses per 10 hpf, often accompanied by some of the following atypical features – increased cellularity, nuclear pleomorphism, solid growth, and necrosis (Fig. 15.51).

- Choroid plexus carcinoma, WHO grade III. These rare malignancies are found in young children. Histologically, choroid plexus carcinoma consists of papillary structures and solid hypercellular sheets of pleomorphic epithelial cells with readily identified mitoses, associated tumor necrosis, and brain invasion (Fig. 15.52). Poorly differentiated examples may be difficult to distinguish from atypical teratoid/rhabdoid tumor.

Fig. 15.52 Choroid plexus carcinoma. This WHO grade III tumor invades the brain parenchyma. It has vacuolated cells and contains foci of necrosis

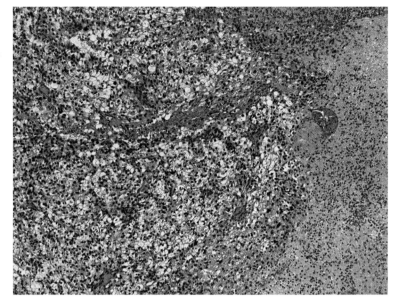

Fig. 15.53 Hemangioblastoma. This tumor is composed of numerous capillaries and sinusoids between vacuolated neoplastic "stromal" cells

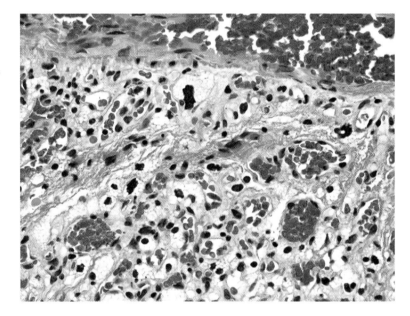

15.8 Hemangioblastoma

This WHO grade I vascular leptomeningeal neoplasm may occur anywhere in the neuraxis but most commonly present as cystic or solid enhancing masses in the posterior fossa. Up to 25 % of the patients with hemangioblastomas have familial (autosomal dominant) von Hippel-Lindau (VHL) disease caused by germ line mutations in the VHL tumor suppressor gene. This tumor consists of abundant capillaries between neoplastic "stromal" cells with round or oval nuclei of varying size, abundant clear or vacuolated, lipidized cytoplasm, and distinctive cellular borders (Fig. 15.53). Occasional stromal cells have giant hyperchromatic nuclei indented by cytoplasmic vacuoles. Mitotic activity is low, and necrosis is rarely seen. Occasionally it may be confused with angiomatous and microcystic meningioma.

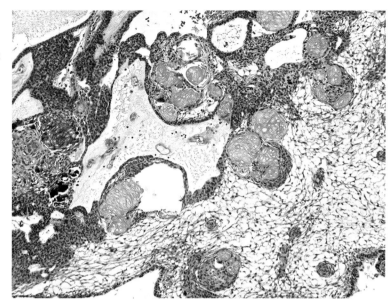

Fig. 15.54 Craniopharyngioma, adamantinomatous type. Strands and islands of stratified squamous epithelium with a prominent "stellate reticulum" pattern and embedded "wet" keratins that calcify focally

15.9 Craniopharyngioma

This WHO grade II tumor typically presents in the form of a circumscribed, often cystic mass in the pituitary fossa and the suprasellar region. It consists of neoplastic, stratified squamous epithelia between supporting stroma that may show old hemorrhage. The epithelia line cystic spaces or form anastomosing sheets with no cytologic features of malignancy. Two morphologic variants have been described – papillary and adamantinomatous. The epithelia in the adamantinomatous variant keratinize and form masses of "wet" keratins that tend to calcify or even ossify (Fig. 15.54). The surrounding gliotic parenchyma often contains prominent Rosenthal fibers.

Acknowledgments The author thanks Dr. Mark A. Edgar at the Emory University for his contribution of Fig. 15.26.

Books and Monographs

Louis DN, Ohgaki H, Weistler OD, Cavenee WK (eds) (2007) WHO classification of tumors of the central nervous system, 4th edn. International Agency for Research on Cancer, Lyon
Love S, Louis DN, Ellison DW (eds) (2008) Greenfield's neuropathology, 8th edn. Hodder Arnold, London

McLendon RE, Rosenblum MK, Bigner DD (eds) (2006) Russell & Rubinstein's pathology of tumors of the nervous system, 7th edn. Hodder Arnold, London
Perry A, Brat DJ (eds) (2010) Practical surgical neuropathology: a diagnostic approach. Churchill Livingstone/Elsevier, Philadelphia

Articles

1. Jansen M, Yip S, Louis DN (2010) Molecular pathology in adult gliomas: diagnostic, prognostic, and predictive markers. Lancet Neurol 9:717–726
2. Mittler MA, Walters BC, Stopa EG (1996) Observer reliability in histological grading of astrocytoma stereotactic biopsies. J Neurosurg 85:1091–1094
3. Daumas-Duport C, Scheithauer B, O'Fallon J et al (1988) Grading of astrocytomas. A simple and reproducible method. Cancer 62:2152–2165
4. McKeever PE, Strawderman MS, Yamini B et al (1998) MIB-1 proliferation index predicts survival among patients with grade II astrocytoma. J Neuropathol Exp Neurol 57:931–936
5. Lind-Landstrom T, Habberstad AH, Sundstrom S et al (2012) Prognostic values of histologic features in diffuse astrocytomas WHO grade II. Int J Clin Exp Pathol 5:152–158
6. Rodriguez FJ, Scheithauer BW, Burger PC et al (2010) Anaplasia in pilocytic astrocytoma predicts aggressive behavior. Am J Surg Pathol 34:147–160
7. Prayson RA, Morris HH 3rd (1998) Anaplastic pleomorphic xanthoastrocytoma. Arch Pathol Lab Med 122:1082–1086
8. Giannini C, Scheithauer BW, Weaver AL et al (2001) Oligodendrogliomas: reproducibility and prognostic value of histologic diagnosis and grading. J Neuropathol Exp Neurol 60:248–262

9. Coons SW, Johnson PC, Scheithauer BW et al (1997) Improving diagnostic accuracy and interobserver concordance in the classification and grading of primary gliomas. Cancer 79:1381–1393

10. Kraus JA, Wenghoefer M, Schmidt MC et al (2000) Long-term survival of glioblastoma multiforme: importance of histopathological reevaluation. J Neurol 247:455–460

11. Kane AJ, Sughrue ME, Rutkowski MJ et al (2012) Atypia predicting prognosis for intracranial extraventricular neurocytomas. J Neurosurg 116:349–354

12. Jeibmann A, Hasselblatt M, Gerss J et al (2006) Prognostic implications of atypical histologic features in choroid plexus papilloma. J Neuropathol Exp Neurol 65:1069–1073

Index

I. Damjanov, F. Fan (eds.), *Cancer Grading Manual*,
DOI 10.1007/978-3-642-34516-6, © Springer-Verlag Berlin Heidelberg 2013